WORKING COPY

BALANCED YOGA

Dr Svāmi Pūrṇá was born into an Indian family of philosophers and rulers. Educated in India and Europe, he later renounced material wealth, position, and possessions. He is a Sanskrit Master and a doctor of medicine, psychology, philosophy, and literature. His mastery of the six schools of Indian philosophy and the Eightfold Path of Yoga have earned him the title Vidya Vacaspati, Lord of Learning.

Dr Pūrṇá's unique courses and seminars on yoga and philosophy have been accredited in the Universities of Europe, the USA and other parts of the world.

BALANCED YOGA

The Twelve Week Programme

Dr Svāmi Pūrṇá

ELEMENT

Shaftesbury, Dorset ● Rockport, Massachusetts

By the same author
The Truth Will Set You Free

© 1990 Dr Svāmi Pūrṇá

First published in 1990 by
Adhyatmik Foundation, Inc

Published in Great Britain in 1992 by
Element Books Limited
Longmead, Shaftesbury, Dorset

Published in the USA in 1992 by
Element, Inc
42 Broadway, Rockport, MA 01966

Cover design by Max Fairbrother
Designed by Vic Giolitto
Phototypeset by Intype, London
Printed and bound in Great Britain by
Billings Ltd, Hylton Road, Worcester

ISBN 1–85230–325–5

Acknowledgements and thanks to
Harriet Bullock D'Agrosa MA, Charlene Dallas,
Petra C Johnson RN, Jane R Pierce RPh, Françoise Rio
and Linda S Spedding PhD
for their editorial contribution
to this book.

CONTENTS

LOOK TO THIS DAY

Look to this day
For it is Life
The very Life of Life
In its brief course lie all
The realities and truths of existence
The joy of growth
The splendour of action
The glory of power.
For yesterday is but a memory
And tomorrow is only a vision
But today well lived
Makes every yesterday a memory of happiness
And every tomorrow a vision of hope
Look well therefore to this day.

KALIDASA

PREFACE

This manual of yoga practice, with its clear illustrations and concise text, is designed to provide expert guidance both to the complete beginner and to the more experienced practitioner of Yoga.

The title *Balanced Yoga* has been chosen to indicate that, while the emphasis is on Hatha Yoga (the yoga of the physical body), you will also find guidance and simple exercises to bring about mental and emotional growth. All in all, the contents of this book will help you to overcome the stressful conditions of modern living, and to promote direction and fulfilment in your life. The programme will enable you to come close to the yogic ideal of a calm and mature mind in a healthy and youthful body.

The lessons are so constructed that each combines physical exercises (asanas), breathing techniques (pranayama), and various relaxation methods with practical concentration and meditation exercises, some thoughts to ponder (including ideas on eating habits), and a few simple disciplines. There is a guiding thought, subject or principle for each week, the physical exercises themselves manifesting this thought, but the selected practices are always balanced so that the whole being may benefit.

This programme is intended as a practical aid. Diligent practice will bring results and will uncover the best in you.

Unless otherwise indicated, all the postures in this book are suitable for both men and women, but if you have any chronic health problem, particularly back trouble, you are advised to consult your doctor before starting this programme.

WHAT IS YOGA?

Yoga is not a religion, a political movement, or dogma. It is a way of bringing harmony within diversity. It respects all cultures, creeds, and nations. It nurtures the higher instincts of humanity – compassion, cooperation, and peace.

It is said that man was made in the image of his creator – healthy, happy, vibrant, and wise – living positively and constantly striving to uplift himself. To be healthy in body and mind, and to be full of vitality, are normal attributes of human life. They are man's birthright. There is little doubt, however, that man has drifted off his intended course. The human mode of living today reflects an attitude which accepts disease and suffering, whether physical, mental, or psychological, as unavoidable and normal. Negative conditioning, habits, and thoughts have thus shortened man's life-expectancy.

Thousands of years ago highly evolved humanists and sages created the system of yoga, a scientific method whereby one is able to develop physically, mentally, and psychologically into a more complete human being. The term 'yoga' is derived from the Sanskrit root *yuk* meaning 'union' or 'yoke'. It implies harmony and balance between all aspects of creation; the impulses and inclinations of the ever-wavering mind being brought under the discriminating yoke of the Higher Self.

Although there are many different forms of yoga practice, the most accessible method for the Western student is that form which takes the physical body as its starting point.

This is Hatha Yoga. The syllables *ha* and *tha* signify respectively the sun and the moon, the flux of positive and negative energies. Balance of these energies results in perfect health, imbalance in disease. Hatha Yoga is thus a complete system of physical maintenance, although physical exercises alone do not constitute Hatha Yoga – that would simply be gymnastics. Hatha Yoga consists of purposefully directed bodily exercises combined with the guidance of the life-force into all parts of the body – each muscle, joint, gland, and nerve fibre – making the body into a conscious and obedient instrument. The combined action of postures with breath control will eliminate poisons and toxins and will vitalize the body, strengthening the whole nervous system. You will begin to feel energetic, yet relaxed. Free from tension, you will be able to cope more easily with the constantly increasing demands of modern living.

However, there is more to Hatha Yoga than a feeling of physical fitness. By stimulating endocrine activity (endocrine secretions being a major component in the 'manufacture' of emotions), Hatha Yoga becomes a valuable aid in the regulation and stabilization of emotion. If practised conscientiously, it will uplift your mind as well as your emotions, it will raise your consciousness, and it will bring you into harmony with the whole of nature. The poet Thoreau expressed it like this:

> Fain would I stretch me by the highway-side
> To thaw and trickle with the melting snow –
> That mingled, soul and body, with the tide
> I too may through the pores of Nature flow.

Interestingly, the word 'Hatha' also translates as 'force' – that tremendous force which you can harness to help overcome many negative manifestations both around you and within you. Hatha Yoga is no self-seeking showmanship, no fanatic asceticism, torture, or fancy gymnastics. It is a scientific tool, pleasant and enjoyable, which can help you achieve balance of bodily, mental, and emotional functions.

About the Postures (*Asanas*)

Lessons are learned from many sources, including the elements of Nature: mountains represent firmness and stability; in rivers we find fluidity and flexibility; trees illustrate the ability of forbearance; and the sun teaches us to shine without expectation or discrimination. The clarity of the sky and the patience of the earth can serve as constant reminders and examples to us.

– Dr Svāmi Pūrṇá

Each creature has attributes or qualities from which one can learn. There is the fearlessness of the lion, the power of the cobra, the alertness of the dog, the industriousness and organizational mastery of ants, the wisdom of the tortoise who withdraws in to his shell, his Self. Birds do not hoard food and they have the ability to fly high. Above all there is the majestic eagle whose strength, power, and endurance enable him to live in surroundings and altitudes unbearable to others. Soaring on lofty wings, he alone enjoys the total freedom of a perfectly clear sky. There is wisdom in contemplating such achievements.

It is said that there are 8,400,000 creatures – and as many yoga postures. Now it is neither possible nor practical for the human being to know and practise even one-thousandth of these. But consider what the mindful contemplation and practice of just a few of those postures could do for you. As you mould your body into a particular pose, directing vital life-force into the corresponding limbs and organs, not only do you exercise and vitalize your whole system, but you also identify with the quality of the posture you assume. For instance, if you perform the balancing posture of a tree for some time, this balance will reflect in your mental and emotional outlook. You are thus building positive qualities into your character.

Although many factors such as environment, people, and past experience will influence you, the results will depend entirely on your own conscientious and steady effort. Hatha Yoga, if practised with purity of body and mind, will enrich the quality of your life.

You must not rush; you must not grow lazy. If your effort is regular and balanced, you will truly enjoy the practice of yoga.

The Breath of Life

Pranayama is the control, regulation, and integration of *prana*, the energy source by which life is sustained. It is sometimes referred to as the 'breath of life'. It is your own energy and that of your environment. As you inhale, you take in air and life energy. Exhaling, you expel the waste products of your body's metabolism.

Today the average person's physical activity has been reduced so much that breathing habits have seriously deteriorated. The body's wonderful breathing apparatus has been so ignored and abused that much of its defence mechanism has become atrophied. Before considering any kind of special breathing exercises, we have to correct any existing faulty techniques and learn to *breathe*.

The air we breathe is designed to enter the human body via the nose. This organ is equipped with fine hairs to filter dirt and dust; it has the ability to moisten and warm the air; and of course it has the sense of smell which warns us of unhealthy, poisonous, or toxic substances. Mouth-breathing in children can have damaging effects which undermine the growth process for life. Tonsils and adenoids become enlarged through having to cope with the onslaught of excessive bacteria, and this often results in the removal of these organs, thereby crippling the child's body defences. Breath intake is often shallow and rapid, giving the lungs no chance to expand fully. Dirt, dust, and germs thus settle easily into the only partially ventilated lungs.

The lack of prana or life-force resulting from inefficient breathing reduces one's natural energy level. To breathe effectively, inhale through the nose, keep an upright posture, avoid highly polluted surroundings such as smoky rooms, and whenever you can during the day, spend a few minutes breathing deeply, fully, and slowly, without straining. Implementation of these few simple instructions alone can bring you renewed energy and well-being.

Breathing is an integral part of each yoga posture. One cannot separate asana from pranayama. The energy taken in with the breath is distributed evenly through the body during the performance of each asana, and the body is thus fortified and the immune system strengthened.

Children and Yoga

Children love to play and impersonate others. To pretend they are a cat, slinking and stretching . . . to sway and move like a tree in the wind . . . to raise up with the silent power of a cobra . . . is tremendous fun for them. Because of the intensity of their identification with the postures, children will quite naturally absorb the appropriate quality and movement. For the boy who pretends time and again to be a lion or hero, fear becomes less likely in situations of his daily life. Likewise, the child who relaxes like a rag doll will fall asleep more easily. Thus yoga will not only help build a healthy physical body for your child, but it will also develop his character.

Much of a child's learning is derived from imitating others, especially their parents. Children follow examples and also absorb impressions from the general environment, so simple postures with inherent positive qualities can become valuable aids in guiding your child's mind and body towards a constructive lifestyle.

A word for those parents whose small children may 'disturb' mother or father's yoga practice: Let them participate. Explain a few suitable postures, maybe tell a little story, and soon they will exercise by themselves. Remember, yoga means 'to join, union, harmony,' and can truly be a great tool to enrich your family life.

BEFORE YOU START YOGA PRACTICE . . .

1. Establish a convenient and regular time for practise; for instance, just after getting up in the morning, or when you come home from work, before dinner, or before going to bed. You will soon discover the time which suits your circumstances best, but please note that if you choose to exercise before going to bed, you should do so more gently than at other times of the day.

2. Before you attempt the exercises in this programme, read right through the relevant chapter so you are mentally prepared for your yoga practice. Where there is a visualization exercise, you may find it helpful to record the instructions on to a cassette, making sure you leave pauses where appropriate.

3. It is important not to have a full stomach. A good guideline is to refrain from eating and drinking for about three hours before practice. However, if necessary you could have a glass of milk or juice. Allow half-an-hour after practice before taking food.

4. It is good to have a warm bath before practice, especially if your body is still a little stiff. Baths should be taken before practice, not after.

5. Wear comfortable or loose clothing. You need to have complete freedom of movement. Do your exercises in bare feet. You may have a pair of warm socks available for relaxation.

6. Use a clean, soft blanket or mat, thick enough to protect your spine and large enough to accommodate your whole body. This blanket or mat should be yours alone.

7. Quiet and clean surroundings with a good supply of fresh air are beneficial. If you have the opportunity and weather conditions permit outdoor practice, do not miss it. It is simply wonderful, especially early in the morning.

8. Privacy – close the door, take the phone off the hook, and make sure you are not disturbed by family

or friends for the time you practise. Your family will soon learn to appreciate the newer, calmer you and will grant you this small request of twenty, thirty, or more minutes by yourself.

9. Before settling yourself on your mat, discard all disturbing thoughts, remembering that nothing is ever improved by worrying about it. You are starting your session in a positive frame of mind.

10. After each yoga session, make a note in a journal or diary of how your body and mind responded to different postures or breathing exercises. Note also any other feelings that may arise.

11. The golden rule of all yogic postures is to perform each exercise slowly, carefully, and mindfully. Force and strain must be avoided at all times. Body mechanics do vary a little from one person to another. There is no competition in yoga – neither with others, nor with yourself.

Once you have completed the basic twelve-week programme, you can continue to use it as your ongoing practice guide. Simply return to the beginning and repeat the course, taking into account your improved flexibility and powers of concentration. In this way, the course can become your lifelong guide.

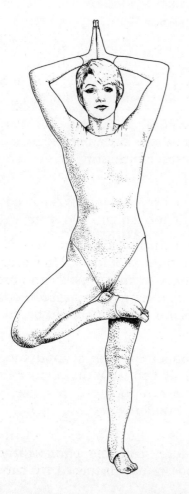

TREE POSE (Vṛkṣāsana)

WEEK ONE

Find a quiet retreat for the practice of Yoga, sheltered from the wind, level and clean, free from rubbish, smouldering fires and ugliness and where the sound of water and beauty of the place help thought and contemplation.

– Śvetāśvatara Upanishad –

Although to follow this advice from one of the oldest yogic scriptures may not be possible for everyone, it gives the general idea that harmonious and serene surroundings are of great benefit. Settle yourself on your mat with crossed legs, and collect your thoughts for a moment. Remember that yoga means union – a harmonious, peaceful relationship with all of creation.

Warming-up

Before you start it is very important to release accumulated tension from various parts of the body. The stretching of muscles and loosening of joints will gently ease you into the programme, bringing you into attunement with your body. The body thus becomes conditioned for the exercises, and you will derive maximum benefit from each posture you perform. Do not be tempted to skip this preparation.

Neckroll

Stand upright. Relax your shoulders. Drop your chin forward and very slowly roll your head across the top of your chest until it eventually comes to rest with your right ear over your right shoulder. After a brief pause, let the head gently drop and roll back across the top of the chest until it reaches a position where your left ear is over your left shoulder. Repeat two or three times. (Avoid turning your face while rotating your head.)

Shoulder and Arm Rotation

Stretch out your arms to the sides, imagining you are between two walls trying to push them apart. Repeat three times. Keep your arms at shoulder level, then rotate the shoulders forwards. Hold for a few seconds. Rotate the shoulders backwards. Repeat three times.

Drop both arms slowly and relax. Observe the sensation this produces in your body.

Gentle Hula

Stand upright, hands on your hips. Gently rotate the hips clockwise in a circular movement three to five times. Repeat the movement in the other direction.

Cleansing Breath

Stand with your feet apart. Inhale fully while you raise your arms above your head in a stretch. Bend at the waist and let your arms fall forward between your legs while you exhale with an open mouth. Repeat three times.

Caution: Avoid this exercise if you have back trouble or suffer from high blood pressure.

Ankle Exercise

Sit down and stretch out your legs. Bending the right leg so that you can reach the foot comfortably, take the right ankle with the right hand. Grasp your toes with the left hand and gently rotate the foot in a clockwise direction three to five times. Repeat the motion in the opposite direction. Take your ankle with both hands and shake it. Repeat the entire sequence with the left foot.

Leg Stretch

Sit with your legs stretched out in front of you. Bend the right knee and grasp the toes (or ankle) of the right foot. Gently straighten the leg. Raise it up as far as is comfortable. Hold while you focus on your leg muscles and let them relax. 'Talk' to them. Bend and relax the knee a little and repeat this stretch twice. Change legs and repeat the sequence. When you are finished, 'shake out' both legs, and lie down and relax.

Spinal Roll

Sit at the foot of your mat with your knees drawn up. Clasp your ankles, make your back round and roll back onto the mat, rocking gently back and forth several times. (A mat or blanket thick enough to protect your spine is most important for this exercise.) Please be careful not to jerk, and beware of rocking too far back onto your neck. Stretch out and relax completely. Observe the effect on your body.

Caution: If you suffer from back trouble you should perform this exercise very gently.

Postures

Swaying Tree

Urdhva Hastottāsana

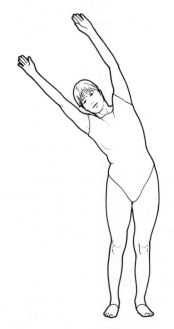

Stand with your feet slightly apart. Raise both arms above your head. Bend from the waist to the right, then to the left, gently swaying to and fro. Repeat five to ten times.

Effect: The Swaying Tree promotes flexibility of the spine, trims the waistline, and relieves constipation.

Cat

Bilikāsana

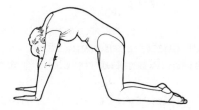

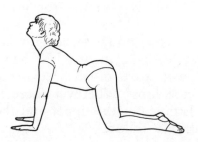

Kneel on all fours with your hands shoulder-distance apart, and your knees the same distance apart as your hands. Your elbows should remain straight throughout the entire exercise. Exhale while arching your back up high. Keep your head between your arms, looking at your abdomen. Hold this pose for a few seconds. Inhale, as you slowly hollow your back to a concave position. Raise your head and look up. Hold again. Repeat the sequence five to ten times, creating a slow, flowing movement of the two postures. Relax and observe.

Effect: The Cat promotes flexibility of the spine. It is good for posture and it strengthens the back and pelvic area. It vitalizes the entire body.

Butterfly

Fatingāsana

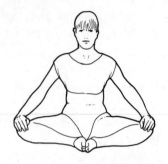

Sit on the floor. Pull both feet towards you, placing the soles together. Grasp the feet with both hands. Gently press the knees to the floor, bouncing them very lightly. Repeat three to five times. Straighten and shake out both legs.

Effect: The Butterfly increases flexibility of the legs and hips, and firms the thighs.

Adamantine Posture

Vajrāsana

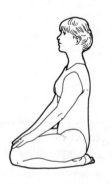

Sit on your heels, knees together, and place your hands on your knees. Breathe slowly and consciously. Slowly raise up on to your knees, keeping your back and head perfectly straight. Sit down in the same manner. Repeat twice.

Effect: The Adamantine Posture is good for knees and thighs. Because it combats sleepiness, it is a good posture to practise after meals as an aid to digestion.

Relaxation *(Savasana)*

Lie down on your mat on your back, your body straight, heels joined, toes apart, and arms alongside the body, palms loosely turned up. Gently close your eyes and mouth.

Focus on your breathing. Remember that the mind and breath are closely connected. By controlling the breath and making it very slow, we are calming the mind. This calmness of mind is essential for good health.

Now relax every limb of your body. Start with the toes by giving them a gentle shake, then relax them. Relax the ankles and lower part of the legs, the knees . . . the thighs . . . the hips. Wherever there is a joint, concentrate on relaxing it – the upper and the lower limbs will automatically follow.

In the same manner, release all tension and tightness in your spine and back. Relax the abdominal area, then relax your chest so the heart and lungs will benefit. Now the shoulders, allowing the relaxation to flow into the arms. Continue on to the forehead to relax the entire face and scalp. The whole body is now completely relaxed. Remain like this for at least five to ten minutes.

Let your breathing be slow and steady, completely rhythmic, and without sound. Then slowly, without jerking or straining, roll on to your right side. Fold the right arm and place it like a pillow under your head. Let heel be upon heel, knee upon knee, the body completely straight, with the left arm loosely placed along your body. You are still relaxed without tension anywhere. Gently roll on to your back. Raise the legs slightly and relax them again. Be sure to keep the entire body straight and without strain. Now turn on to the left side and repeat the procedure. Gently roll back on to your back. After taking a deep breath, exhale slowly and sit up with ease.

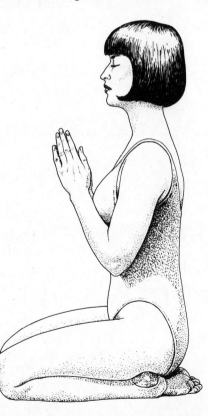

ADAMANTINE POSE (Vajrāsana) with Respectful Greeting (Namaskar)

Effect: Relaxation following the exercises is a process in which no active tension is generated in the muscles of the body. During the state of profound relaxation, muscle tension and intra-tissue tension fall drastically. This results in an increased blood-flow into the tissues, providing the muscles with nutrients and oxygen essential for releasing energy. At the same time, waste products are being washed out of the system.

It is believed that the feeling of fatigue after exercising is due to accumulated waste matter. The speedy disposal of waste results in relief from fatigue. It is essential to conclude each practise session of yoga asanas with total relaxation.

Discipline and Practice

It is recommended that you practise these postures regularly, preferably every day. During the coming week, make an effort to walk and move gracefully, in a relaxed manner, rejecting thoughts of strife, anger, or dislike. Remember that you are part of the Whole and so are others.

WEEK TWO

The first fruits of the practice of Yoga are: Health, little waste matter, and a clear complexion, lightness of the body, a pleasant scent and a sweet voice – and an absence of greedy desires . . .

— ŚVETĀŚVATARA UPANISHAD —

That quote is encouraging. Of course, one cannot expect all the above results after one week's practice. However, even in such a short time many new students will already have experienced an increased feeling of well-being, freshness, and vitality. These are the results of the cleansing process that has been set into motion.

Most people already have a simple routine of daily hygiene, such as bathing, cleaning their teeth, and so on. A useful addition to your mouth care can be the cleaning of your tongue. Have you noticed that in the morning your tongue may be thickly covered by a greyish coat? This is just another of the body's mechanisms for removing toxins and harmful bacteria; yet unless you remove these deposits, they will simply be re-ingested with your food and drink. Make cleansing your tongue part of your morning routine. You can do this by gently 'scraping' your tongue with an inverted teaspoon, which will remove most of the coating. (Keep the same spoon and store it with your toothbrush.) Your mouth will feel fresh and clean, appreciating the taste of wholesome food.

Focus on Peace

Sit on your mat in an easy, cross-legged posture, hands resting on your knees. Scan your memory for an experience that conveyed much peace and serenity to you. This may be a walk by the sea . . . a few moments in a majestic forest . . . a sunrise in the mountains . . . a sunset across a limpid lake . . . anything which brings back the silent beauty and peace of the moment. Recall the feeling of peace without dwelling too much on the actual incident. Let peace flood your mind and body, leaving your entire being in a state of serenity.

Warming-up

Woodchopper Swing

Stand straight, with your feet about two feet apart. Inhale, raising your arms straight above your head. Bend backward as far as is comfortable. Hold. Exhale, slowly swinging forward and down through the legs. Inhale . . . and repeat the sequence twice. Relax and observe.

Caution: If you suffer from back trouble, you should avoid this exercise until you feel your back has begun to loosen up and strengthen through regular yoga practice.

Ankle Exercise

Refer to Week One.

Leg Stretch

Refer to Week One.

Leg Lifts

Lie on your back, with your arms spread out at shoulder level. Bend the left knee (to prevent back strain), foot on the floor. Raise the right leg as far as is comfortable, keeping the knee perfectly straight. Pull your toes toward you. Hold for three to five seconds. Lower your leg slowly as you exhale. Repeat twice. Change legs and repeat the sequence with the other leg. Then raise both legs together. Hold for three to five seconds. Gently lower both legs together, exhaling as you do so. Be sure to keep your knees straight throughout the exercise. Now relax and observe your body.

Effect: Leg lifts are most beneficial for strengthening the abdominal muscles and lower back.

Caution: If you have lower back problems or sense any undue strain in this area, you may wish to bend the knees slightly as you raise and lower your legs.

Spinal Roll

Refer to Week One.

Postures

Cat

Refer to Week One.

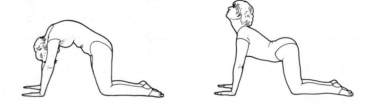

Pelvic Twist

Ardha Vakrāsana

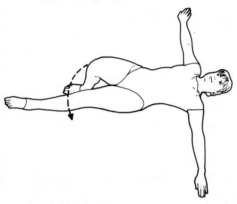

Lie on your back, arms stretched out at shoulder level. Bend the right knee, placing the right foot beside the left knee. Lay the right leg to the right side. Then bring the right leg across the body to the left side, touching the knee to the floor. Return the knee to an upright position. Straighten the leg. Now repeat the sequence with the left leg. Relax and observe.

Effect: The Pelvic Twist promotes flexibility of the spine and hips. Good for minor spinal adjustments, it promotes equilibrium of energies in the body.

Cobra

Bhujaṅgāsana

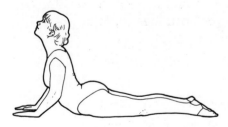

Lie face down. Place the palms on the floor under the shoulders, fingers turned slightly inward. Slowly lift the forehead, the nose, the chin, and the entire upper body, up to the navel. The weight rests on both hands, the pelvis, and the legs. Keep the elbows slightly bent, and do not allow the shoulders to hunch up towards the ears. Hold for ten seconds, focusing your attention on the lower back. Very slowly lower your trunk to the floor, then the chin, the nose, and the forehead. Relax and observe your body.

Effect: A posture of prime importance, the Cobra increases the influx of blood into the abdominal organs, relieves indigestion, constipation, and flatulence, and has a similar stimulus to the spinal region, so the body is completely revitalized. The Cobra prevents and corrects spinal deformities and is indispensable for the correction of kidney malfunctions, such as recurrent infections and the formation of calculi (stones). It is good for those with a slow thyroid function, and it also promotes confidence.

Caution: To be practised very gently. Avoid this asana if you have a tendency to hernia.

Child's Pose

Vajrāsana Variation

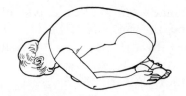

Sit on your heels. Slowly bend forward, allowing the forehead to rest on the floor, arms lying loosely by your sides. Hold and relax into this pose for as long as is comfortable. Lift up slowly, unrolling the body, raising the shoulders and the head last.

Effect: Relaxation. The Child's Pose stimulates the circulation in the extremities and the head. It is good for all the abdominal organs, combats fatigue, and promotes humility.

Inverted Pose

Viparita Karani

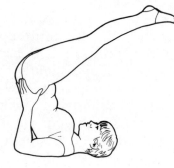

Lie on your back. Slowly raise your legs off the floor. Supporting your hips with both hands, bring your legs slightly over your head. Straighten both legs and remain in this position for as long as comfortable. Focus on your face and throat. Very slowly lower both legs. You may bend the legs coming down if necessary.

Effect: Rejuvenation. The Inverted Pose increases circulation in the neck and face and is a natural 'face-lift'. Both the heart and the lungs benefit. The Inverted Pose is also good for varicose veins and haemorrhoids.

Caution: This posture, in common with other inverted postures, should be avoided if you suffer from high blood pressure, hyperthyroidism, or heart trouble. It should also be avoided during heavy menstrual flow.

Tree Pose

Vṛkṣāsana

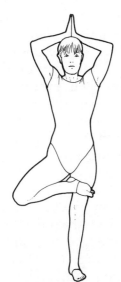

Stand with both feet together, arms loosely by your sides. Focus your eyes on an imaginary spot directly in front of you. Bring the right foot up and place the sole against the inside of the left thigh, as high as possible. When balanced, raise both arms simultaneously, placing the palms together over your head. Hold for thirty seconds. Gently lower your arms. Release your foot from your thigh. Repeat the sequence with the other foot. When you are finished, relax and observe your body.

Effect: This is a concentration exercise, promoting balance and stability of body and mind.

Complete Breath

Lie on your mat, face up, arms lying loosely by your side. Gently close your eyes and mouth. For a few moments observe the rhythmic ebb and flow of your normal breath. Then place your hands lightly on the area around your navel.

Exhale slowly, emptying your lungs as completely as possible. Do not force. Now inhale slowly through the nose, gently pushing out the abdomen, then expanding the rib cage, and finally raising the upper chest and shoulders as you complete the inhalation.

At the end of the inhalation you will notice a slight retraction of the abdomen. This is the beginning of exhalation. In the same order, exhale through the nose as you tighten the abdomen, then contract the ribs, and finally relax the shoulders.

Inhalation and exhalation should follow each other smoothly and easily in a wave-like pattern. Determine your own pace.

This technique may require a little practice. Make certain to avoid any kind of strain in your breathing.

Relaxation

Now you are ready for relaxation. Remain lying on the floor and continue to breathe slowly and naturally.

Focus on your feet. For a moment give your feet your undivided attention. Now let go and relax them. Feel the feet tingle and become warm and heavy. Focus on your ankles and relax them . . . calves . . . knees . . . thighs . . . concentrating all your attention on each part in turn, then releasing and relaxing. Your legs will now feel warm, heavy, and comfortable.

In the same manner, focus on your buttocks for a moment . . . and let go. Bring your attention to the spine. Starting with the lowest vertebra, let your focus slowly travel up the entire length of the spine, right up to the neck. As you let go and relax, notice that your entire back is relaxing, that it is free of tension and feeling warm and comfortable.

Now bring your attention down to your abdomen, concentrating especially on the area around the navel. As you let go and relax, feel the warmth and comfortable weight of your internal organs. Move your attention to your chest, and as you relax feel the heart pump more slowly and the lungs ventilate more slowly.

Focus now on your neck and shoulders and, as you relax, feel any remaining tension from the neck and shoulders drain out through the upper arms, lower arms and hands, and out through the fingers . . . leaving your arms and shoulders comfortable and relaxed.

Concentrate on your throat. Swallow once or twice. Move your attention to your face, relaxing your chin, cheeks, nose, eyes, ears, and forehead in turn. As you relax your forehead, the scalp also relaxes.

Your entire body now feels relaxed, warm, and heavy. As you remain in this posture for some time, the body may begin to feel lighter, and you may perceive a pleasant floating sensation. Do not concern yourself with thoughts that may enter at this time. Remain peacefully relaxed for at least five to ten minutes.

As you come out of the relaxation, take time gently to 'awaken' your body. Move your hands and feet first, take a deep breath or two, stretch your arms above your head, and stretch and tense your whole body for a couple of seconds. Then gently roll on to each side in turn (as in the relaxation exercise of Week One) and finally sit up gently.

Discipline and Practice

During the coming week, contemplate on the effect of focused thought, its choice and intensity. Giving any thought your attention helps it grow. A negative thought will grow just as much as a positive one – and can affect you accordingly. Be mindful of the kind of thought you are seeking and nurturing. Such censorship of thought can become an invaluable aid in the practice of emotional stability.

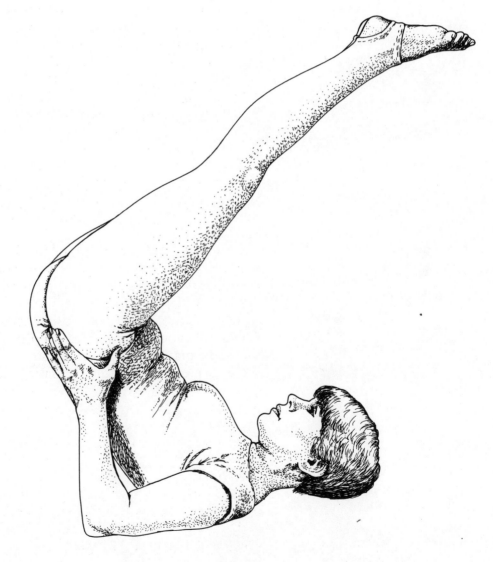

INVERTED POSE (Viparita Karani)

WEEK THREE

To gain, preserve and utilize life energy are the three aspects of the physical body's power.

– DR SVĀMI PŪRṆĀ –

Both the quality and the quantity of life energy are determined by the intake of food, water, and air, as well as by the elimination of waste products and by thought and emotion. Anger, jealousy, or hatred actually create poisonous substances within every cell; whereas love, kindness, and compassion have a healing, soothing, and regenerating effect on the body. Day by day we build ourselves by what we eat and drink, by the air we breathe, and by our mental processes. Contemplation on this can teach us that every day we have a choice: to build or destroy.

Postures and breathing exercises for this week have been chosen to help with the elimination of waste matter and the building of body and mind.

Focus on Peace

Sit on your mat in an easy, cross-legged posture, hands resting on your knees. Relax briefly, closing your eyes and calming your mind. Breathe easily and naturally. Recall an experience of peace and serenity. Let the peace of the memory flood your mind and body, leaving your entire being in a state of serenity.

Warming-up

As in Week Two.

Postures

Swaying Tree

Refer to Week One.

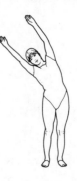

Mountain Pose

Parvatāsana

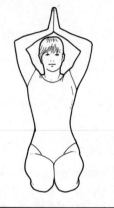

Sit on your heels or with crossed legs, holding the body very straight. Raise your arms above your head, placing the palms together, and inhale, using the complete breath technique. Exhale while lowering your arms to your knees. Repeat twice.

Effect: Good for respiratory ailments, the Mountain Pose also increases determination and resistance.

Raised Serpent

Nāgāsana

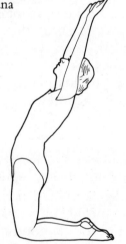

Sit on your heels, knees together, and place your hands on your knees. Slowly raise yourself into a kneeling position while lifting your arms above your head. Lean back while keeping the body straight. Hold for as long as is comfortable.

Effect: The Raised Serpent increases resistance and builds willpower. Excellent for weak knee joints.

Triangle Pose

Trikoṇāsana

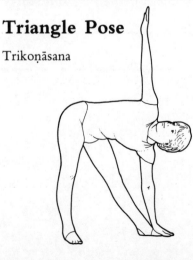

Stand with your feet about three feet apart. Inhale and raise your arms sideways to shoulder level. Turn your left foot ninety degrees to the left and your right foot forty-five degrees to the left. Exhale and bend from the waist to touch the left foot with the left hand. The right arm points up, forming one straight line with the left arm. Turn your face towards the upraised hand. Hold for ten seconds. Inhale and return to a standing position. Turn your feet to the right in the same manner and perform the exercise on the right side. Repeat twice more to each side – slowly, smoothly, and carefully. Relax . . . and observe.

Effect: The Triangle Pose is unique in restoring the equilibrium of the nerves. Toxins are eliminated, and boils, pimples, and many infections are prevented. General good health results. The Triangle Pose is also good for lung ailments and back problems like lumbago and sciatica. The body becomes light.

Locust Pose

Śalabhāsana

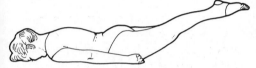

Lying face down on your mat, rest your head on your forehead. Keep your arms alongside the body and make your hands into fists. Inhale and raise both legs,★ keeping the knees straight. Hold for ten seconds. Exhale and slowly lower the legs. Relax and repeat twice. If you find this exercise too strenuous, you may raise one leg at a time until you can raise both comfortably.

★Although these instructions suggest you raise your legs on the inhalation, some people in fact find it easier and more comfortable to perform this movement on the exhalation. Decide for yourself which you prefer.

Effect: This is a good posture for everyone. It stimulates digestion, relieves constipation, and has a profound preserving effect on the kidneys. The spine and entire back are strengthened.

Note: Practise of this posture affects the finer tissues and smaller blood vessels in the back. Just as locusts have a distinctive and highly developed faculty of 'hopping high', this asana sublimates many of the human being's baser faculties.

Caution: Do not attempt the Locust if you suffer from high blood pressure.

Wind Liberating Pose

Pavana Muktāsana

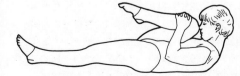

Lie flat on your back. Inhale. Exhale and pull up your right knee toward your chest with both hands. Bring your head and knee together. Hold for ten seconds. Inhale and straighten your body. Change legs and repeat the sequence twice. Relax and observe.

Effect: Relieves the accumulation of gas in the intestines and improves digestion. The Wind Liberating Pose imparts lightness to the body.

Inverted Pose   Refer to Week Two.

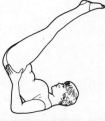

Breath Control

Cleansing Breath

Three times. Refer to Week One.

Complete Breath

Do seven rounds. Refer to Week Two.

Complete Breath with Chin Lock

After a complete inhalation, hold the breath while pressing the chin firmly against the chest for about ten seconds. Release the chin as you exhale slowly. Perform three rounds.

Effect: Builds willpower.

Relaxation

Fear is one of the most destructive emotions. It causes stress, and stress causes disease. Here is a simple but effective method to overcome fear.

After relaxing your body in the usual manner, step by step, touch the centre of your chest with your fingertips and place your consciousness there. Fear will instantly leave you.

Discipline and Practice

'You are what you eat.' Whatever you eat or drink you make a part of yourself. Anything you take into your body becomes an integral component of you, influencing you on all levels – physical, mental, psychological, and spiritual. Different foods, all varying in their attributes, produce different chemical reactions in the human body.

Take a look at what is being offered on today's market. Do we choose a certain food because it looks attractive, because it tastes good? Do we also consider the healthful and nutritive value of the food we select?

The purpose here is not to go into details of what to eat and when – countless books are available on this subject – but simply to help you become aware of your eating habits. Developing discrimination between foods that build and maintain the body, and those substances which pollute the system and hasten the ageing process, can prevent the premature breakdown of the body. When the body is full of metabolic impurities, the mind will be equally affected.

Unspoiled, natural food is available throughout the year. Keeping in mind that the seven essential nutrients for good health are proteins, fats, carbohydrates, vitamins, minerals, roughage, and water, and by applying a little mindfulness in the selection of groceries, nutritious and balanced meals that are also very tasty can be produced. The practice of offering resistance to unhealthy or undesirable external influences will not only increase your body's resistance to illness and stress, but also strengthen your mind and character. You really *are* what you eat.

During the coming week, keep vigil on your dietary habits, take note of your likes and dislikes. Examine to see if they are supportive of health and well-being, of inner cleanliness, or if your senses often overrule your common sense.

Hint: Do not eat when angry or upset. You will only feed the emotion, and your anger will grow.

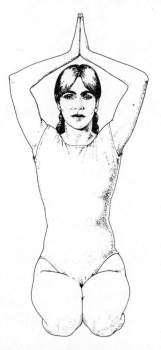

MOUNTAIN POSE (Parvatāsana)

WEEK FOUR

When the body is in silent steadiness, breathe rhythmically through the nostrils with a peaceful ebbing and flowing of breath. The chariot of the mind is drawn by wild horses. These horses have to be tamed.

– ŚVETĀŚVATARA UPANISHAD –

It has already been mentioned how vital it is to breathe correctly. Your entire energy is influenced by the way you breathe, and so too are your thought processes. Breath and mind are closely related and affect each other continuously. Notice how anxiety is accompanied by shallow and rapid breathing; and how, by the same token, it is possible to calm the agitated mind through conscious rhythmic breathing. Breath control provides one of the most effective tools against stress and anxiety in today's life of hectic activity.

There are many techniques which specialize in building the heart and lungs to capacity so these organs will know no exhaustion. Yogis are able to increase the amount of oxygen they take in, and can manage to exist quite efficiently and energetically with whatever limited amount of oxygen the atmosphere affords. In this way they can live in areas where air is rare, such as on the Himalayan summits, twenty-two thousand feet above sea level. With this amount of control, they are also able to prolong their lives.

Proving or achieving the miraculous is not important, but such examples can provide understanding of the full capabilities of healthy human breathing. Poor breathing technique and a stunted breathing apparatus will eventually result in disease.

This week's exercises have been selected to help you develop and strengthen your breathing potential and to relieve such conditions as chest congestion, chronic catarrh, even asthma.

Focus on Peace

Briefly relax and focus on peace.

Warming-up

Neckroll
Refer to Week One.

Shoulder Rotation
Refer to Week One.

Triple Bandha
Bandhas are 'locks' wherein certain body areas are contracted and tightened.

Rowing: Sit on your mat, legs stretched out in front of you. Now visualize yourself pulling the oars of a rowboat. Lean forward, arms outstretched and exhale. Inhale as you pull and lean back. Press your chin tightly against your chest, with the abdominal and anal muscles tightened. Repeat forward and backward movements about seven times.

Cauldron: Remain in the same position with your legs stretched out in front of you. Imagine yourself stirring a giant cauldron as you move your arms in a large circle. Do seven circles in each direction.

Bell Pull: Sit with your legs stretched out in front of you. Inhale and raise your arms high above your head. Visualize holding a heavy rope with both hands to pull a heavy bell. Exhale and pull down slowly with all your strength. Perform seven times.

The practice of the above exercises can stimulate your energy level considerably. The Cauldron and the Bell Pull movements will promote the circulation in the lungs and heart.

Please do relax and rest after these exercises and observe the effect they have on your body.

Leg Lifts
Refer to Week Two.

Postures

Simple Twist

Vākrāsana

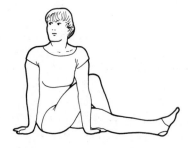

Sit with outstretched legs. Pull the right leg towards the body. Place the right foot across the left leg on the floor, next to the left knee. Inhale. Twist the upper body to the right, placing both hands on the right side of the body on the floor. Look over the right shoulder and exhale. Hold for at least ten seconds. Inhale as you slowly move out of the posture and repeat on the opposite side. This posture is very gentle and is easily performed.

Effect: The Simple Twist strengthens the entire nervous system and helps overcome spinal deformities. The crossing of the positive and negative currents (*ha* and *tha*) affects their equilibrium and results in perfect health. Psychologically this posture induces balance, stability, and self-confidence.

Cobra

Refer to Week Two.

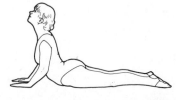

Head-to-Knee Pose

Māha Mudrā

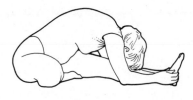

Sit with the right leg stretched out. Flex the left leg and place the sole of the foot against the right thigh. Inhale, raising both arms. Exhale and slowly lower the body to grasp the right foot with both hands. Rest your head on the right knee. Repeat the posture very slowly, and then perform twice on the other side. Take care to move into and out of this posture very carefully and smoothly. Relax and observe.

Effect: The Head to Knee Pose unifies solar and lunar energies within the body, promoting balance, resistance, and immunity. It increases lung capacity and removes odours from bodily secretions. The higher instincts in the human being are awakened.

Cow-Face Posture

Gomukhāsana

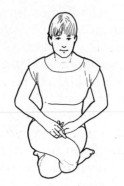

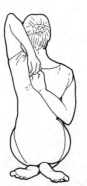

Phase One: Sit on the floor, legs stretched out in front of you. Bend the left leg, placing the left heel on the outside of the right hip. Lift the right leg over the left leg, with the right heel touching the outside of the left hip. Note how the arrangement of the feet resembles the shape of a cow's or bull's horns.

Effects: The currents of *ha* and *tha* are crossed, promoting equilibrium within the body, and a calm balanced mind. This pose stretches and brings elasticity to the sciatic nerve. Regular practice brings much relief from the painful condition of sciatica.

Note: Only attempt the Cow-Face Posture if you are fit and healthy. You may find that you have to persevere with your general yoga practice before performing this exercise.

Phase Two: Sitting in the above pose with the right leg on top, raise and bend the right arm to touch the middle of your back. Reach back with the left arm from waist level and grasp the fingers of the right hand. Keep your head and neck erect. Hold for at least ten seconds. Repeat the pose on the opposite side, changing the positions of your legs to place the left leg on top, and raising the left arm to touch the middle of the back.

Effects: The Cow-Face Posture stimulates development of the arms and shoulders. It is of great benefit in lung diseases, since the respiratory movement of the lungs is alternately arrested and increased. This asana is a powerful cleanser for the alveoli of the lungs.

Inverted Pose

Refer to Week Two.

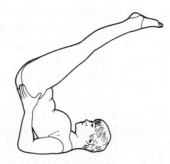

Holy Fig Tree Pose

Asvattāsana

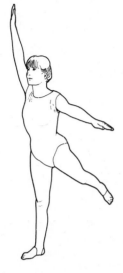

Stand upright. Raise your left arm upwards, your right leg backwards, and your right arm out to the side. Hold. Release and perform on the opposite side.

Effect: Although so simply performed, the benefits of this pose are remarkable. It promotes the circulation of prana, the vital life-force within the entire body, resulting in increased oxygen absorption and a greater release of carbon dioxide. The Holy Fig Tree, or Pipal Tree, is considered a superior kind of tree, since it continues to release oxygen even at night. In this posture the energy level is raised, respiratory problems are eased, and blocked nostrils are freed. It is also good for allergies. Excellent during pregnancy, it improves foetal blood circulation and alleviates labour pains.

Relaxation and Breath Control

Lie down and relax in the usual manner. When your body is quite relaxed, turn your attention to your breath. Begin by breathing slowly, evenly, and deeply. Exhale and imagine yourself expelling all the poisons and waste products of the metabolism, together with any negative thoughts or ideas. When you inhale, visualize that you are being filled with pure, healing energy, that you are being revitalized and renewed.

Discipline and Practice

An old legend informs us that when the Creator gave the gift of life to the human being, he also gave him a certain number of breaths. Once these were used up, the individual would have to leave his body . . .

In view of such economics, contemplate how rapid, shallow and irregular breathing is related to negative emotions, compared to the blissful infusion of energy resulting from peaceful, equalized breathing.

During the coming week, make a point of getting out and about for walks, taking in fresh air, especially early in the morning. If living in the city, you could use the city park or spend a day out in the country. You may not have any Holy Fig Trees in your neighbourhood, but trees in general provide oxygen and vital life-force. They are also soothing to the eye, inspiring to the mind, and a delight to the soul.

WEEK FIVE

Discipline is the essence of yoga – discipline of the body and discipline of the mind.

— Dr Svāmi Pūrṇá —

Discipline of body, mind, and emotion is essential to a well-integrated and fulfilling life. Lack of self-control creates anxiety, fear, and stress. A few well-directed disciplines will result in less hardship than that caused by desire and lack of self-control. Discipline can help you strengthen your sense of resolution and willpower, thus channelling your energies in a more positive direction.

A trained and disciplined mind becomes a reliable servant. A mind driven by desire and directed by its own impulses turns into a tyrannical master.

Focus on Peace

Briefly relax and focus on peace.

Warming-up

As in Week One.

Postures

Forward Bend (Standing)

Pādáhastāsana

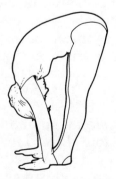

Stand straight, the feet slightly apart. Inhale, raising your arms above your head. Exhale, slowly bending forward from the hips and place your hands on the floor next to your feet. Gently push your head towards your knees. Hold for a few seconds. If you find it difficult to touch the floor, bend forward as far as comfort permits and hold your legs just below the calves. Straighten up very slowly by 'unrolling' your body as you inhale again. Repeat only once.

Effect: The Forward Bend is a unique posture that revitalizes the spine, the nervous system, and all the abdominal organs. The increased blood circulation to the brain results in relief of fatigue and better concentration. The inner ear also benefits, thereby correcting disturbances in the sense of balance, and many other latent dysfunctions in the body are eliminated. Additionally, the shoulders are strengthened, the waist becomes slim, and weight loss is initiated.

Caution: Please do not push or strain beyond your limits. Avoid jerking or bouncing at any time.

Note: If you suffer from duodenal ulcers, high blood pressure, or low blood pressure, you should practise the following modified version of the Forward Bend:

Stand straight, feet slightly apart. Place your hands round your waist, pulling your shoulders and elbows back. Inhale and raise your chin three or four inches. Exhale and slowly bend forward from the hips until your trunk is parallel with the floor. Do not bend any further forward, and keep your chin raised throughout. Hold for a few seconds and then slowly return to the starting position as you inhale. Repeat once.

Hero

Virāsana

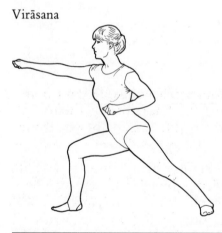

Stand straight with your arms by your sides and your feet about three or four feet apart. Turn your body and the right foot about ninety degrees to the right. Bend the right knee, stretching the left leg. Push the right arm forward and pull the left arm back, angled sharply at the elbow. Make your hands into fists. Hold for at least ten seconds, breathing normally. Release the pose and repeat, bending the left knee. Relax and observe.

Effect: This asana will strengthen your feet, thighs, knees, and arms, and reduce the waistline. The Hero combats lethargy, and imparts strength, courage, fearlessness, fortitude, and power.

Lion

Simhāsana

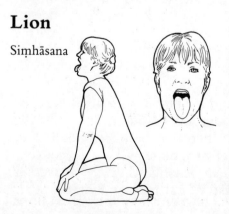

Kneel on the floor and lower your body to sit on your heels. The arms are locked straight with the hands pressed against the knees, fingers spread open. Inhale. Open your mouth as much as possible and push out your tongue as far as you can, touching the chin. Exhale forcefully. Relax. Repeat at least five times.

Effect: Although not the most graceful pose, this asana is second to none for curing a sore throat in a hurry, often within minutes. The voice becomes clear, bad breath is eliminated, teeth and jaws are strengthened, and eyesight is improved. Continued practice helps to overcome stammering. This asana also generates fearlessness, gives the 'energy of a lion', and engenders more self-controlled behaviour and response.

Caution: Avoid this exercise if you suffer from heart trouble or high blood pressure.

Finger Balance

Tolaṇgūlāsana

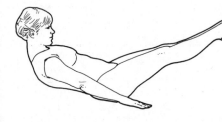

Lie flat on your back, arms by your sides with the palms facing downwards. Raise your legs and upper body simultaneously, balancing on your buttocks. The arms are stretched forward with the fingertips touching the floor. Hold for a few seconds and gently lower your body to the floor. Repeat twice. Relax and observe.

Effect: This asana is invaluable for those who wish to increase their willpower, resistance, and balance. Nervousness is overcome. This asana is also helpful when feeling cold, as the body becomes warm.

Caution: Be particularly careful with this exercise if you suffer from low back problems.

Shoulder Stand

Sarvaṇgāsana

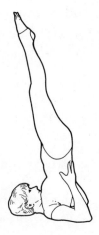

Lie on your back with your arms alongside your body. Slowly raise your legs off the floor, lifting them back over your head. Continue to lift your hips and trunk, supporting your hips with your hands as in the Inverted Pose. When you are steady and comfortable in this position, raise your hips further up, moving your hands up your back until the body is in a straight line, or as far as you can, with feet pointing toward the ceiling. The chin is pressed firmly against the chest, and your body now rests on the shoulders, the nape of the neck, and the upper arms. Relax into this position by breathing slowly, using your abdominal muscles.

When first practising this posture, remain in the most upright position for a few seconds only. Gradually you may extend the time spent in the Shoulder Stand.

Caution: Do not practise this asana if you suffer from heart disease, hyperthyroidism or high blood pressure. It should also be avoided during heavy menstrual flow.

Effect: The reversal of the gravitational flow in the body effects a regeneration of the entire bodily system. Especially good for the spine and abdominal organs, the Shoulder Stand posture also has a cleansing and strengthening effect on the throat, tonsils, eyes, and sinuses. It prevents greying of the hair, removes body odours, and counteracts fatigue. The increased venous blood return makes it invaluable for those who suffer from varicose veins and haemorrhoids.

The Fish

Matsyāsana

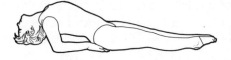

Lie on your back, both legs stretched out, feet together. Raise the upper body and rest on your elbows. Arch your back and bend your head backward until the crown of your head touches the floor. Hold for a few seconds.

To come out of this posture, lift your head and gently lower the body to the floor. Please be careful not to stretch or strain the neck. Repeat once or twice. Relax and observe how your body feels.

Effect: The Fish is of great benefit to the eyes, thyroid, throat, and lungs, and is also good for colds and lung ailments. The upper spine is strengthened.

The extended neck of the Fish posture is the natural counterpose after the Shoulder Stand's extreme pressure on the neck.

Breath Control
Complete Breath

Sit on your mat with crossed legs and a straight back. Breathe rhythmically through your nose as explained in Week Two. Continue for about three minutes, relaxing into the posture and letting your breath flow evenly. Do avoid any kind of strain or force.

Chin Lock

Jálandhara Bandha

Remain in a cross-legged position. Exhale fully, and then inhale fully, without strain. Now hold your breath while pressing the chin firmly against your chest for a few seconds. Lift your head and exhale slowly. Repeat two or three times.

Effect: The Chin Lock increases willpower.

Relaxation

Relax your body step by step as in Weeks One and Two. When completely relaxed, repeat mentally a positive affirmation to help you increase willpower, resolution, perseverance – or whichever quality you feel you need to develop most. Here are some examples:

'My performance is improving daily.'
'I work with enthusiasm and continuity.'
'What I set out to do I complete.'
'My willpower is growing daily.'
'I persevere in my task through all difficulties.'
'My body is strong, my mind is firm.'

If you wish to choose your own words, befitting your situation, make sure your statement is a positive one, 'I have . . . I do . . . I can . . . ' This is accepted far more readily by the subconscious mind than a negative statement.

Discipline and Practice

A simple and constructive discipline for gaining some mastery over the senses is the control of speech. Much time and energy are wasted in idle talk – even more in malicious gossip or verbal abuse. Gossip can be a most destructive mental and emotional poison, doing great harm to both perpetrator and victim.

Speech energy can be used wisely in uplifting and inspiring conversation, in words of solace, courage, and truth – and in silence. Unless there is a useful and constructive comment to be made, why speak at all? It has been said that he is wise who knows that he has nothing to say, and cannot be persuaded to say it.

During the coming week, observe your speech habits. Are they constructive, pleasant, firm? Do your words impart comfort, trust, cheerfulness, encouragement, and help to others? Or does your speech portray vagueness, manipulation, even aggression? Do you say things you later regret? Contemplate the wisdom of this ancient Arabian proverb:

Blessed is he who speaks a kindness,
Thrice blessed is he who repeats it.

WEEK SIX

He who is moderate in food and movement, in his engagement in actions, in sleep and wakefulness, attains to yoga – which destroys misery.

– BHAGAVAD GITĀ –

Last week we spoke of discipline as the essence of yoga. However, even the most excellent discipline, carried to an extreme, can distort into fanaticism or self-torture.

Observe a pendulum. Note how it swings to and fro off its centre-line. The physics of the pendulum hold one of the most valuable lessons of life. As you push the pendulum in one direction, it will swing out, return to baseline, and then swing in the opposite direction in a compensatory movement. Your whole life has the characteristics of a pendulum. Thoughts, words, and actions determine the intensity of its swing – and its compensatory return to the opposite pole.

If you overwork, you will experience exhaustion. If you loaf all day, the evening will find you restless and discontented. Overindulgence in the pleasure of eating will be followed by the pains of indigestion – not to mention the scales. People whose moods and emotions swing from extreme joy and hilarity to the depths of grief and depression are considered 'unbalanced'. Life's pendulum is too active for them. When emotional balance is disturbed, it creates a stressful influence on the entire system. You react, instead of thinking and analysing in a calm manner; and by reactions, once again, the pendulum is set in motion. Before jumping into anger, pause and think awhile. Endeavour to control your emotions, or they will control you. Life will constantly present its ups and downs, its peaks and valleys. Skilful and contented living requires the peaks to be smoothed down a little and the valleys to be filled a little. If great joy does not overwhelm you, pain and sorrow will find you equally stable. Balance is one of the greatest teachings of yoga.

Each week the selection of asanas and pranayama is balanced to affect the whole body. This week's programme has been carefully chosen so that the performance of each posture will help to establish the equilibrium of your physiological energies, and to raise your ability to bring thought, emotion, and habits into a more harmonious and balanced relationship.

Focus on Peace

Briefly relax and focus on peace.

Warming-up

Basic Stretch

Stand upright, feet together. Inhale and raise your arms, stretching as far as possible. Exhale and lower your arms. Repeat five times.

Swaying Tree

As in Week One.

Waist Rotation

Still standing, spread your arms out at shoulder level. Slowly and smoothly twist from the waist to the right, then to the left. The lower part of the body remains still. Breathe in rhythm with your movements. Repeat five to seven times in each direction.

Cat Stretch

As in Week One.

Leg Lifts

As in Week One.

Leg Lifts with Space Walk

Raising both legs, as above, perform a walking movement in the air for about thirty seconds, keeping the knees straight and the toes pulled towards you. Gently lower your legs. Relax and observe.

Postures

Simple Twist

As in Week Four.

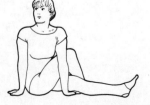

Lion's Pose

As in Week Five.

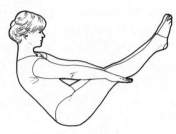

Crescent Boat

Nāvāsana

Lie on your back, arms lying loosely by your side. Inhale. As you exhale, raise your legs and upper body simultaneously, balancing on your buttocks. Raise both arms and stretch forward horizontally, fingers pointing toward the knees. (If necessary, hold knees with both hands.) Hold the posture for a few seconds. Slowly lower your body to the floor. Repeat twice. Relax and observe.

Effect: The whole body is balanced and strengthened, and the spine is revitalized. The energy centre around the navel becomes aligned, correcting digestive disturbances and regenerating all abdominal organs. Nervousness is overcome and the body becomes warm.

Caution: As with the Finger Balance (Week Five), you should approach the Crescent Boat with caution if you suffer from low back trouble. It would be advisable to strengthen your back through regular yoga practice before attempting this exercise.

Swing Posture

Dōlāsana

Lie face down and stretch your arms above your head. Inhale and simultaneously raise your arms, upper body, and legs. Hold for ten seconds. Exhale and relax on the floor. Repeat twice. Relax completely and observe.

Effect: The whole body is revitalized, and posture is improved. Good for digestion and abdominal 'flab'. Also good for lungs and circulation. The body becomes light and agile. Willpower and resistance are heightened.

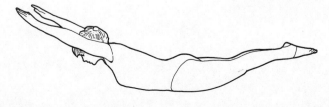

Ox Posture

Vriṣabhāsana

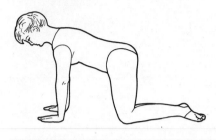

Kneel with both hands on the floor. Breathe smoothly and evenly. Turn your feet to the right for one minute, then to the left for one minute.

Effect: A very easy posture for most, the Ox Posture induces a feeling of well-being, tranquillity, and steadiness of mind, and also brings relief from flatulence. While the feet are turned to the right, the left nostril becomes free; the right nostril becomes unblocked when the feet are turned to the left.

Plough

Halāsana

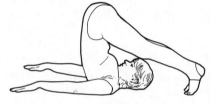

Lie on your back, arms by your sides, palms down. Slowly raise your legs and trunk (as in the Inverted Pose, Week One). Keep the legs as straight as possible. Supporting your back with both hands, continue lifting your legs and trunk up and over your head until the toes come to rest on the floor behind your head. Should you notice excessive tension in your back, spread your feet apart the first few times you do this posture. Only when you are quite comfortable in the position, release the hold on your back and place your arms flat on the floor. Hold only for ten seconds in the beginning. After your body becomes accustomed to this position, you may hold it longer. Very slowly unroll your body to the starting position.

Effect: Wonderful for the entire nervous system, the Plough results in instant removal of fatigue, listlessness, and exhaustion. It corrects spinal deformities and affects the regeneration of the chest, lungs, and all abdominal organs. It is of particular benefit to diabetics, due to its regulating effect on the pancreas and endocrine glands.

Caution: Please do not practise this asana if you have a spinal disc lesion.

Tree Pose

As in Week Two.

Breath Control

Complete Breath

(With acceleration and deceleration.) Sit upright in the usual manner and breathe rhythmically, as in Week Two. After about one minute, very slowly increase your rate of breathing just a little and for a few seconds only, then slow down again for a few seconds. Continue for a total of two or three minutes.

Effect: Balance.

Alternate Nostril Breathing

Again sit upright with your spine erect and your head level. You may find it helpful for concentration to close your eyes. Using your right hand for this exercise, fold the index and middle fingers into the palm, leaving the thumb, fourth, and fifth fingers free. The thumb will control the right nostril, and the fourth and fifth fingers will control the left nostril. Proceed as indicated:

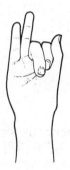

Close the right nostril with the thumb and inhale slowly and fully through the left nostril.

Hold for two or three seconds only. No longer.

Close the left nostril with the fourth and fifth fingers and exhale slowly through the right nostril.

After a natural pause, inhale through the right nostril while the left nostril is still closed.

Again hold for two or three seconds only.

Close the right nostril and exhale through the left nostril.

This completes one round. Beginners should limit themselves to three rounds. Rounds may be increased as your system adjusts.

Effect: Balance and equilibrium in both body and mind. Alternate nostril breathing also purifies the nerves, and brings relaxation and refreshment.

Tips To Help Your Balance

If balancing postures have been a source of frustration to you, the following ideas may help to correct the difficulty.

First of all, check your technique. When performing the Tree Pose, for instance, ensure that the hips are level and that the suppporting foot, the tailbone, and the neck are in direct alignment. Visualize the supporting leg 'pushing' into the floor.

Inhale deeply as you raise your arms above your head, and concentrate your gaze on a spot in direct line with your eyes. The breath should be calm and even. Do not force concentration as this will impart rigidity to your body and create further imbalance.

Forcing balance on your body while in a state of emotional upheaval will also prove frustrating; in fact, it will increase the difficulty. However, if you can acknowledge your emotions and current limitations, you can begin to deal with them. Laughing at your own temporary ungainliness or at a tumble may solve the problem then and there. Worry, anger, and emotional upset are often accompanied by a feeling of constriction and of tightness around the navel and heart region. Heartfelt laughter can bring noticeable release almost instantly, re-establishing equilibrium.

Most of you have experienced situations of illness, grief, and other upsets, times when 'leaning' on another person for a while provided the support which enabled you to find your own balance – to stand on your own two feet again. By the same token, you can use a temporary support for your balancing postures. Use a prop such as a chair, the wall, or anything you can hold on to briefly for support. The mere pleasure and satisfaction of being able to do the posture will eliminate much frustration and will promote further improved balance.

You cannot, of course, lean against or hold on forever to a wall, a chair, people, ideas, institutions, or habits. Props are tools designed to help you find your own balance within your own self-reliance.

Relaxation and Meditation

The Flower Garden

Relax the body, step by step. Breathe slowly and rhythmically. Quieten the mind by letting all your thoughts float away like clouds in the sky. As you begin to enter the silence of your being, visualize a beautiful garden. Let it be all you wish it to be.

Entering the garden, notice that there is a place where you may leave all the burdens you are carrying with you . . . the worries . . . the anger . . . the frustrations of the day . . . any thoughts that are keeping you from being totally free and happy. Place them in the space reserved for you.

Now look around and notice all the different glorious flowers. Find one that particularly attracts you and sit down in front of it. Look at it, touch it, notice how it feels, inhale its fragrance. Ask it to share its essence with you.

Now let your essence blend with that of the flower . . . feel yourself as the flower. Notice how you feel being rooted in the ground, how the wind sways you in its breeze . . . notice the warmth of the sun . . . Feel your skin become as the petals and let yourself be bathed in the flower's perfume.

As the sun begins to set, become aware of the evening breeze, the appearance of the stars, the brightness of the moon and the healing stillness of the night . . .

With the breaking of dawn, feel the dew on your petals and merge into the poignant stillness of Nature . . .

Now the sun rises. Thank the flower for sharing her essence with you. Saturate your being with the perfume of the flower and the feeling of oneness you have experienced. Gradually become aware of your body again. Know that you may return to this communion with the flower at any time.

Become aware of your breathing, of your body lying quietly, and slowly begin to move your fingers and toes. Stretch your arms above your body, and tense your body briefly. Then turn on to your right side, then slowly on to your left side, and finally roll slowly on to your back once more. Open your eyes when you are ready.

Discipline and Practice

Patanjali, a great logician of ancient times, states in his treatise on the science of yoga, *The Yoga Sutras*, that ' . . . meditation is the unbroken flow of thought towards the object of concentration.' In other words, whatever you may concern yourself with or think about intently, whatever you concentrate upon, you enter into, make a part of yourself, and gain knowledge thereof. Such is the law.

Thinking is a serious responsibility. Using this process consciously, remember that you determine the choice of the object of your concentration and subsequent meditation. It is unwise to underestimate the risk of persistent, haphazard thought.

A constant flow of thought towards ugliness, violence, or crime, or towards incidents and objects which arouse negative emotions such as anger or jealousy, is not likely to result in serenity and contentment. It will create fear and misery. However, to let the mind dwell on truth, beauty, and goodness will have an uplifting and wholesome effect upon your whole system. The flower meditation you have just done will illustrate this point.

In the ensuing week you may wish to contemplate on further wonders of Nature . . . on the majesty of an ancient oak tree . . . on the purity of freshly fallen snow . . . on the magnificence and serenity of a sunset over a quiet lake . . . Let your imagination take you on a peaceful walk through the forest or by the ocean. Any experience or situation which affects you peacefully and serenely is of benefit. When meditating on Nature, you identify with the nature of Nature and all her manifold aspects. You also perceive the perfect balance and harmony which prevails in Nature – despite the efforts of humankind to upset this balance.

The process of meditation is a wonderful tool to gain balance and strength in meeting the difficulties and temptations of life. It can transform your life. Take a moment to reflect on the relationship between the concentrated performance of asanas, thought discipline, meditation, and your own evolvement. Then meditate in solitude, and in quiet, peaceful surroundings. Meditate on love, tolerance, forgiveness, strength, and patience. Meditate on the perfect balance in Nature, and on the perfect balance within your own body and your own being. And one day, you may wish to go beyond body, beyond Nature . . .

WEEK SEVEN

Surya Namaskar: The Salute to the Sun

O life-giving Sun, offspring of the Lord of Creation, solitary seer of heaven! Spread thy light and withdraw thy blinding splendour that I may behold thy radiant form: that Spirit far away within thee is my own inmost Spirit.

— ISÔPANISHAD —

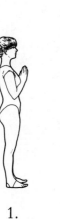

1.

2.

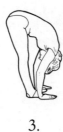

3.

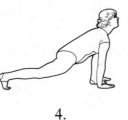

4.

5.

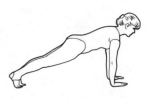

6.

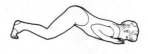

7.

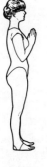

12.

11.

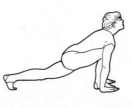

10.

9.

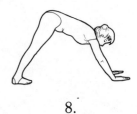

8.

Long before the age of technology, the forces of Nature were worshipped. People felt reverence for the life-sustaining qualities of the sun, moon, trees, oceans, rivers, and other aspects of Nature. Nations throughout the ages have attributed the status of divinity to the sun, for our planet could not survive without its light and warmth. In harmony with the myths of ancient sun-worshippers, modern technology not only acknowledges the value of solar rays, but, in view of the constantly dwindling supplies of earth's energy, it looks with hope and reverence towards a future powered by the inexhaustible supply of the sun's energy.

Even this gigantic heavenly body is itself powered by the great Cosmic Source, as is each individual being. We are all individual rays of the Source, and it shines freely through us when we are not limited by our own self-imposed barriers. As mind and body become lighter, more purified, and more subtle, the body can be permeated with energy that is received, held, and used in uplifting activities.

Focus on Peace

Briefly relax and focus on a peaceful moment you have experienced.

Warming-up

As in Week Six.

Postures

The Salute to the Sun

The Surya Namaskar, or Salute to the Sun, has evolved from a beautiful combination of asanas, pranayama, mudras (gestures), and contemplative meditation. Like the sun, it has twelve divisional components. The twelve postures flow smoothly into each other, and involve and affect every part of the body and the mind. Ideally, it should be practised in the open air each morning at dawn, facing the rising sun.

Effect: Every part of the body is influenced. The chest is broadened, the arms are beautified, and dermatological disorders are prevented or corrected. It stimulates digestion, helps to relieve abdominal complaints such as constipation and congestion, and reduces the tummy or paunch. Its practice makes the spine and waist flexible and it relieves lethargy. In keeping with the sun's characteristics of light and brightness, the Salute to the Sun is the natural 'anti-depressive'.

Caution: It is not advisable to practice the Salute to the Sun after the third month of pregnancy, nor if one suffers from extremes of low or high blood pressure, or from hernias. Also, if you suffer from back trouble, it is advisable to strengthen your back through regular yoga practice before adding the Salute to the Sun to your programme.

To achieve the greatest benefit from the Salute to the Sun, perform the movements conscientiously and allow the breath to follow each posture as described below. Each posture should be held for several seconds.

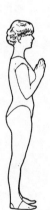

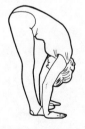

1. Stand erect, feet together, hands together in front of your chest, in a prayer pose.

2. Inhaling slowly, stretch the arms up and back, tightening the buttocks and bending backwards as far as possible.

3. Exhaling, bend forward, touching the forehead to the knees (or as far as possible) and placing the hands flat on the floor in front of the feet. Keep both knees straight.

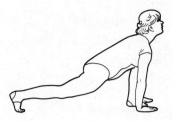

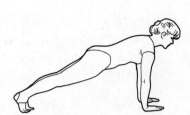

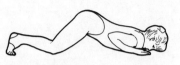

4. On the inhale, place the right foot as far back as possible, toes touching the floor. Keep the palms on the floor in the same position. The head is up.

5. Exhaling, bring the left foot back to meet the right one. Hands and toes are touching the floor. Head, back, and legs form a straight line.

6. Holding the breath, turn the hands in slightly and bend the arms and knees so that the toes, knees, chest, hands, and forehead are touching the floor.

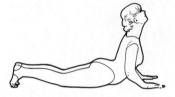

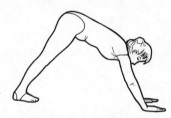

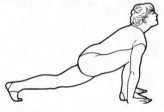

7. Inhale and straighten the arms, bending backwards, the lower body resting on the floor.

8. Exhale while raising the buttocks off the floor. The hands and feet remain flat on the floor, making the body an upside down 'V'.

9. Inhale, bring the right foot forward, knee to chest, and raise the face upward.

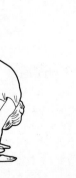

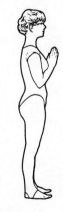

10. On the exhale, bring the left foot up, level with the right one. Keeping the legs straight, touch the forehead to the knees.

11. Inhaling, raise the hands up and behind the head. Bend backward, tightening the buttocks.

12. On the exhale, bring the hands together in front of the chest, fingers pointing up in the prayer pose, looking straight ahead.

The Salute to the Sun should always be done in pairs, one round beginning by placing the right foot back, and the second round beginning by placing the left foot back. Two rounds comprise one cycle. Perform two cycles, and then lie down for several minutes to observe and enjoy the benefits of the exercise. This exercise has a highly invigorating effect on both body and mind, and can be practised alone as a complete 'mini-routine'.

Relaxation

Complete step by step, as in Week One or Week Two.

There is a beautiful mantra for greeting the sun:

OM NAMO SURYAYA

OM NAMO BHASKRAYA

OM NAMO DIVAYA

OM NAMO TEJAYA

OM NAMO PRKASHAYA

OM NAMO SURYAYA
I recognize the sun within me; it is the cause, the source of my life. It is the energy that flows through me.

OM NAMO BHASKRAYA
It is the sustenance sparkling into every cell of my body – vital energy spreading throughout, new rays incessantly beaming into me.

OM NAMO DIVAYA
It is my source of nourishment; it creates new life in me.

OM NAMO TEJAYA
It promotes brightness and vitality in me.

OM NAMO PRKASHAYA
It enlightens me, fills me with knowledge, dissolves darkness. I invoke the sun, source of my life. I will place you, Sun, in my body so it may function fully, to the last cell.

A mantra is not a prayer nor a religious hymn, but a technique by which one can increase one's own energy. It is a method of psychosomatic healing. Whether or not one understands the Sanskrit terms is not so important; the sounds will still have the desired effect. Certain 'seed' syllables have within them the power to affect nerves and glands, and these 'seeds' can be planted deep within the psyche by repetition, for the assistance of growth. Mantra Yoga is an entire form of yoga based on sound therapy.

The sun mantra may be spoken at sunrise or at sunset, or you may wish to repeat the mantra during the performance of the Sun Salutation – after you have thoroughly familiarized yourself with the postures. Alternatively, you may repeat it silently during relaxation.

WEEK EIGHT

As the sun that beholds the world is untouched by earthly impurities, so the Spirit that is in all things is untouched by external sufferings.

— KATHÔPANISHAD —

It is said that for those who really want to learn, the whole world becomes a university. Consider the sun further. What can be learned from this great fiery orb whose daily light and warmth we generally take for granted?

Constantly, without discrimination, this powerful dispenser of life energy sheds its rays on everything alike, remaining equally unaffected by splendour and squalor. Each human being, microcosm of this gigantic energy system, has a solar plexus for the reception and distribution of cosmic energy. The solar plexus is a network of nerves and blood vessels lying between the ribs and the abdomen. Energy, cosmic and otherwise, is said to enter the body at this point. Often much of this energy is depleted through insignificant mental and physical activities, negative thinking, and purposeless conversation. Loss or waste of energy exhausts your 'powerhouse' and results in disease and misery. However, the energy that is held, preserved, and wisely directed will engender physical health as well as mental, psychological, and spiritual growth. Systematic and economical use of energy is a secret of the yogis.

If your personal energy level is low, this week's programme can help you to correct this deficiency. Remember, though, that the type of food you eat also plays a large role in your energy level. Fresh and raw foods contain a great deal more prana than dishes in which cooking has destroyed much of the life-force.

Focus on Peace

Briefly relax and focus on the peace within you.

Warming-up

Cat Stretch
As in Week One.

Leg Lifts

As in Week One.

Leg Stretches

As in Week One.

Ankle Exercise

As in Week One.

Knee Limbering

Sit on your mat with your legs stretched out in front of you. Bend the right knee and place the right foot on the left thigh, as close to the groin as is comfortable. With your fingertips, gently push the right knee toward the floor about ten or fifteen times. Repeat this exercise with the left leg.

Please be gentle with yourself. Do not force for any reason. Many knees are very stiff and it takes time and practice to loosen these joints.

Postures

Mountain Pose

As in Week Three.

Swan

Haṇsāsana

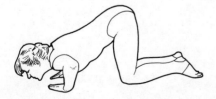

Kneel, with both hands on the floor, knees about one foot apart, and the hands slightly turned inward. Inhale. While exhaling, bend the elbows and lower the chin to the floor. Inhale and move the body forward in a gliding movement, keeping the chin close to the floor. Exhale and 'glide' back to the starting position, still keeping the chin close to the floor. Repeat twice.

Effect: The Swan is a most effective asana for strengthening the chest, shoulders, and the often neglected wrists. It strongly affects the solar plexus and the energy centre of the heart. The Swan aids determination and concentration, and also imparts gracefulness and the impetus to overcome obstacles.

Forward Bend

Paschimottānāsana

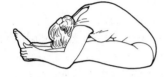

The leg lifts and stretches you have performed during the warming-up period are considered an essential preparation for this asana.

Sit with your legs stretched out in front of you, knees very straight. Inhale and stretch your arms above your head. Exhale and very slowly and smoothly bend forward from the hips (*not from the waist*) to grasp your toes. If at first this seems difficult, clasp instead your ankles, calves, or knees. It is important that your legs remain quite straight. Continue to bend forward and down, aiming to touch your knees with your head. Hold for at least ten seconds and observe your breath. Release your hold and very slowly unroll your spine, returning to a sitting position. Repeat twice.

Note: This asana may require diligent practice to perform in its perfection. Practice will also help you to develop patience. Never force your body; never bounce or jerk. Rather let your body slide and relax into the posture.

Effect: Until a few decades ago, this Forward Bend was considered a yogic secret and was never performed in public. It is said that by virtue of this posture and its inherent control of pranic life-force, yogis can prolong their lives indefinitely.

This may be stretching your yogic aspirations, but we have already mentioned the close relationship between the rate of breathing and the human life span. During the performance of the Forward Bend the body requires less oxygen, and the respiratory rate is slowed down by about fifty per cent in the average human. Both the slow breathing and the steady pressure exerted on the solar plexus will restore balance to an overactive and excitable state of mind.

Other benefits include vitalization and increased suppleness of the spine, relieving lumbago and sciatica. Heavy thighs and buttocks are reduced. The blood circulation in the whole body is stimulated, and the abdominal organs are regenerated, thereby improving digestion. It is good for skin disorders and also removes body odours.

Pelvic Stretch

Suptá Vájrásana

Kneel on the floor and lower your body to sit on your heels in the Adamantine Posture as in Week One. Place both hands behind you, fingers pointing away from you. Slowly raise the pelvis and trunk into a nice arch, looking upward, and keeping your seat on your heels. Hold for ten seconds. Return to the Adamantine Posture. Repeat twice. Relax and observe the effect on your body.

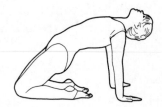

Effect: The Pelvic Stretch is very good for posture and for relieving tension in the body. All the major joints benefit. It is excellent for respiratory ailments and is a basically stimulating exercise.

Note: Occasionally, after forward and backward bending, some slight discomfort may be experienced in the lower back. This can easily be relieved by lying on your side, head cradled on bent arm, and raising the top leg for a few seconds. Turn on to the opposite side and repeat.

Tortoise

Kūrmāsana

Again kneel in the Adamantine Posture. Bend your arms and place your elbows against your navel area, with your hands made into fists. Bend forward to rest your face on your knees while pressing your elbows into your navel area. Hold for ten to twenty seconds, release, and return to the Adamantine Posture. Repeat twice. Relax and observe your body.

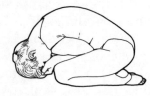

Effect: The Tortoise is a very simple asana which generates heat and increases metabolism. It raises the energy level by activating the 'fiery sun chakra' – the energy wheel situated around the navel area. This posture has a strong regenerative effect on the liver, pancreas, and adrenals. It aids concentration and introspection. Like the tortoise who withdraws into its shell, this asana enables people to detach themselves from unwholesome and negative external conditions as well as from unwanted mental and sensual associations.

Simple Twist

As in Week Four.

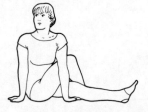

Half Lotus

Ardha Padmāsana

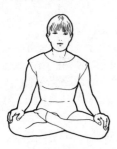

The knee-limbering exercises of the warming-up routine are an essential prerequisite to this posture.

Sit on the floor with outstretched legs. Bend the right knee and place the right foot against the groin – the knee rests on the floor. Bend the left knee and gently place the left foot on top of the right thigh, as close to the groin as you comfortably can. Straighten your back so that your trunk, neck, and head are in a direct line.

Your hands may be placed in either of the following positions:

1. Resting on your lap, palms up, with one hand resting in the other. You will notice your body feeling lighter.

2. Resting on your knees, palms upturned, with the thumb and first finger joined in the Lotus Mudra (gesture). You will notice your body feeling heavier.

Close your eyes and relax into this pose for as long as you are comfortable. Slowly release and gently shake your legs.

Performing the exercise on the opposite side, you will often find that one side is more comfortable than the other. Discover which one is most suited to your body and practise that one regularly.

Effect: Having overcome the initial discomfort in the knees, the Half Lotus can be a most comfortable and relaxing pose. Posture is improved, the digestive and reproductive systems are strengthened, and mental discipline and concentration are also improved.

Breath Control

Complete Breath

Do seven rounds.

The Bellows

Bhastrika

This pranayama is an exception to the smooth, gentle, rhythm usually performed in breath control exercises. Bhastrika literally means 'the bellows', the tool a blacksmith uses forcibly to blow air into the fire. Similarly, The Bellows breath raises the heat of the body by stimulating the fiery sun *chakra* (see p. 00), thereby fuelling all bodily systems. It is a highly cleansing and invigorating exercise and should only be performed in a healthy body.

Stand with feet about one foot apart. Bend your knees slightly and rest your hands on your thighs. Very slowly and almost imperceptibly begin to breathe through your nose – in and out. Gradually and smoothly increase both the rate and depth of your breathing until the breath rushes in and out deeply and rapidly. At the point of exhaustion, STOP. Lie down immediately in the Relaxation Pose (savasana). This is the most sensitive moment of the exercise, the point at which your thought process can change direction.

Caution: Never attempt The Bellows if you suffer from abnormal blood pressure or heart disease.

Effect: The performance of The Bellows brings an additional blessing to those who struggle with unwanted thoughts. In the presence of this fire, an old thought can be 'burnt up', to be replaced by a new and healthy thought. Determine the choice of your new thought at the beginning of the exercise.

Relaxation

It is wonderful to go straight into complete relaxation after the above exercise, incorporating the candle visualization described below.

Discipline and Practice

Humans have the ability to be like the sun and to reflect the great Cosmic Light in all their dealings and behaviour. However, we generally have preferences – we like certain things, places and ideas, and dislike others; we favour one person but reject another. Unfortunately this kind of discrimination enforces the illusion of separateness, which is counter to growth.

There is a simple technique for radiating light and love into the environment:

Candle Visualization

Place a lighted candle before you and concentrate on its flame for some time. Let your body relax, breathe evenly, and gaze steadily at the flame . . . After a few minutes, close your eyes and visualize the flame and its aura in the centre of your chest, its radiance spilling out beyond the confines of your body . . .

Once you are able to visualize the candle's flame without the candle actually standing in front of you, you can incorporate projecting its light while you are in deep relaxation.

Effect: Through practice you can develop this ability 'to shine', creating a healing and soothing effect on those around you as you influence your environment by your own positive energy. Do you ever have the urge to improve the world but do not know how? By becoming this flame, this constant positive energy field, you will do the greatest service to the world, to your family and friends, and to yourself.

WEEK NINE

When man becomes steadfast in his abstention from harming others, all creatures will cease to feel enmity in his presence.

– YOGA SŪTRAS –

By this aphorism Patanjali expresses the principle of non-violence, of *ahinsa*. This is the essence of yoga, of union, of integration, and the realization that all is one. Ahinsa requires us to live in such a way that no other creature is harmed by our thoughts, words, or actions. Patanjali's statement speaks of energy, the high vibration of pure harmlessness, readily and instinctively perceived by all creatures.

The meaning and extent of harm caused by action towards plants, animals, and fellow humans is sadly apparent all around us. Verbal violence manifests in abusive, foul language, slander, and gossip. Yet the most elusive form of injury is through thought. Thought is less tangible, apparently fleeting. Thoughts of anger, hatred, envy, resentment, and jealousy all contain the element of harm toward others. Such projections of negative thought energy reflect on the individual's surroundings by producing reactions like antipathy and fear. Thoughts of intended harm promote the arousal of instincts for self-preservation – flight or fight – and vital energy is thus depleted.

The conscious practice of ahinsa, however, has wonderful results. Energy previously wasted in the three forms of attack can now be stored. Stored energy converts into power, which is cumulative, and you become a 'powerhouse of positivity'. The high vibration of genuine harmlessness, of selflessness, compassion, and love transmits itself to all beings. A shield of absolute positivity renders aggression harmless. This is the power which conquers all.

Focus on Peace

Relax briefly and turn your attention to a place of peace within you.

Warming-up

Stretching and Reaching

Stand upright and raise both arms above your head. Stretching your entire body, reach out and up with each hand alternately, about ten or twelve times. Relax by letting the upper body fall into the woodchopper swing.

Leg Stretch

As in Week One.

Butterfly

As in Week One.

Cat Stretch

As in Week One.

Knee Limbering

As in Week Eight.

Postures

Salute to the Sun

As in Week Seven. Perform one cycle.

Action Pose

Karmāsana

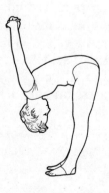

Stand upright, feet together. Clasp your hands behind your back and exhale. Keeping your hands clasped, inhale and raise your arms up and back as high as possible, pinching your shoulder blades together. Bend forward from the hips, keeping your back quite straight. Now lift your chin. Make sure that your legs are straight. When you are comfortable in this position, continue to bend forward, exhaling, bringing your head as close to the knees as is comfortable. Hold for ten to fifteen seconds. Slowly unroll and return to a standing position. Repeat twice. Relax and observe your body.

Effect: The Action Pose is a wonderful revitalizer for those who experience periods of sluggishness during certain times of the day. Stale air is emptied from the lungs, and the influx of fresh air and improved blood circulation promote an increased flow of vital life-force into the upper body. You will feel instantly refreshed and able to continue concentrated work.

Note: If you suffer from duodenal ulcers, high blood pressure, or low blood pressure, you should practice the following modified version of the Action Pose:

Stand upright, feet together. Clasp your hands behind your back. Inhale and raise your chin three or four inches. Exhale and bend forward from the hips, keeping your back straight and your shoulders pulled back. Stop as soon as your trunk is parallel to the floor. Keep your chin raised. Hold for ten to fifteen seconds. Inhale and slowly straighten up. Repeat twice, then relax and observe your body.

Bow Pose

Dhanūrāsana

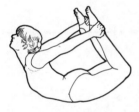

Lie on your mat, face down, arms by your sides. Bend the knees and reach back to grasp both ankles. Take a couple of normal breaths. Inhale and slowly raise your head, upper body, and legs off the floor. Visualize your arms being the string which pulls up the bow of your body as your body rests on the waist and abdomen. Breathe normally and hold for about ten seconds. Very slowly lower the body to the ground and release the legs. Repeat once more. Relax completely and observe the changes in your body.

Effect: The Bow is often called the anti-ageing pose, due to its pronounced effect on the endocrine system. The stimulation of the gonads (sex glands) postpones the onset of menopause and old age. The pose is highly beneficial to diabetics due to the stimulation of the pancreas and increased release of insulin. It is also good for those suffering from thyroid deficiency and slow comprehension. There is a general toning of all the abdominal organs. The spine becomes resilient, posture is improved, and the cause of many backaches is removed. This posture is a wonderful general preventative against disease.

Please perform this asana very slowly and gently. To heighten the effect, gentle rocking may be added.

Caution: Do not practice the Bow Pose if you have over-activity of any of the endocrine glands or a tendency towards hernia. (Check with your doctor.) The Bow should also be avoided in the second half of pregnancy, and for six months after an abdominal operation.

The Half-Twist

Ardha Matsyendrāsana

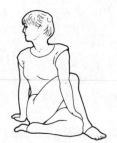

The Simple Twist you have performed many times will have prepared you for the next stage. Sit with both legs stretched out in front of you. Bend the left knee and place the left foot against the groin. Take the right foot and place it across the left leg on the floor, at the outside of the left knee. Turn your upper body to the right and place the right hand behind you on the floor. Lift the left arm over the right leg and grasp the right knee. Look over your right shoulder and relax into the pose, breathing slowly. Release the pose gently and perform on the opposite side.

Effect: The resultant balancing of negative and positive energies leads to general harmony and good health. It is an excellent posture for spine and hip joints, and is also good for chronic ailments of the abdominal organs, especially the liver, spleen, and pancreas. Conscientious practice of this asana can arouse latent powers and abilities.

The Plough

As in Week Six.

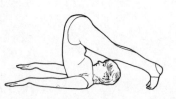

Rishi's Pose

Rishiāsana

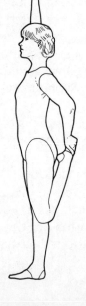

Stand upright with your feet together. Shift your weight on to the right foot. Bend the left leg and grasp the ankle behind you with the left hand. Press the ankle close to the body. Check your balance: hips should be level, tailbone in line with both the right heel and with the neck. Push the weight-bearing foot 'into' the floor. Inhale and raise your arm above your head. Look straight ahead – do not look at your upraised hand, as this will upset your balance. Breathe normally and hold the pose for as long as is comfortable. Repeat the pose with the opposite leg.

Effect: Rishi's Pose improves physical and mental balance. It gives poise to posture, stretches the upper thighs, and promotes concentration.

Breath Control

Complete Breath

Perform seven rounds.

Sitali

Sit comfortably, preferably in the Half Lotus or the Adamantine Pose. Shape your tongue into a tube and push the tongue through O-shaped lips. Inhale, drawing the air over the curled tongue. Hold your breath for three to five seconds and exhale slowly through the nose. Repeat five times.

Effect: Effectively cools the body and relaxes the nervous system. Very good during fevers because of its cooling effect and the elimination of toxins and poisons. Sitali also improves the complexion.

Relaxation

Beautiful Meadow

Visualize yourself walking through the countryside. It is a warm and sunny day. Your path winds slowly through a meadow – the most beautiful meadow you have ever seen. The grass is like a luscious carpet, dotted with wild flowers that gently waft in the warm breeze. The air is filled with the scent of flowers and the rich aroma of the warm earth.

Let yourself relax and stretch out in the soft, fragrant grass. You inhale deeply, feeling contentment and a sense of belonging. All is well . . . all is in order . . .

Looking around, you notice a bee busily gathering honey from a clump of purple flowers. A ladybird struggles up a stem of grass, falls off, and begins to climb another stem. Somewhere near you a lark starts up and flies into the air, warbling its song. Your eyes follow the little bird as it climbs higher and higher into the blue sky, singing its song to Nature and its Creator. Now the lark is only a tiny speck in the sky, and as it climbs higher still, that too is lost to the eye. Yet, listening very carefully, you can still hear the lark's song of praise.

Puffs of white cloud are drifting across the clear, blue sky . . . Visualize your thoughts as puffs of cloud and see them drifting by, one by one, vanishing into the distance, leaving your consciousness to merge with the endless blue sky . . . widening . . . extending . . . expanding . . . (Allow yourself an extended pause here.)

Slowly let your awareness return to your body lying in the grass; then let the scene slowly fade from your consciousness. Bring your attention back to this room and to your body lying on the floor. Begin to move your hands and feet, take a few deep breaths, and stretch your body well. Open your eyes and sit up when you are ready.

Discipline and Practice

Ancient sages have stated that the real test of ahinsa is in the absence of jealousy. One should be as enthusiastic about the success of others as one is about one's own. During the coming week, focus on your feelings if someone moves into a space that you had previously considered yours. Examine the feelings that this arouses in you. How do these emotions affect you? Do they arouse thoughts of rivalry, of aggression? Can you remain neutral toward the 'rival'? Can you maintain kind, loving thoughts?

> *Let not the arrow in thy hand*
> *Hurt man or any living being;*
> *Let it be an arrow of love.*
>
> — SVETASVATARA UPANISHAD —

WEEK TEN

Humility is born of the knowledge that all is ONE; it demands profound respect for life-producing Nature.

— Dr Svāmi Pūrṇā —

As you diligently continue on the path of yoga, your health, strength, and vitality may increase to such an extent that it greatly surpasses the energy level of those around you. There may also come a stage when these reawakened latent energies will manifest as a power you have not experienced before. This power is intriguing and elating. Suddenly you begin to realize the more profound aspects of yourself. Unfortunately, many stop at this point, caught by ego and pride. Thoughts of being special, of becoming powerful, will retard your progress. This is the opposite of yoga, which means harmonious integration with all of creation.

Contemplating the *source* of your newly-found energies will help you to escape the trap of pride and ego. True growth is reflected in humility rather than pride. Be humbly grateful that you have discovered the means towards greater happiness and fulfilment, and work on it every day.

Focus on Peace

Relax briefly and focus on the peace within you.

Warming-up

As in Week One.

Postures

Crocodile

Makarāsana

Lie face down on your mat and stretch your arms above your head. Stretch the entire body and hold for ten to thirty seconds.

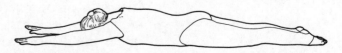

Effect: This asana is considered an exception, as it is the only one whose effects are opposite to the behaviour of the creature it depicts. The Crocodile generates a submissive, humble, and reverential attitude. The body is made strong, straight, and firm, and the respiratory rate is reduced.

Bowing Down Pose

Bhūmāsana

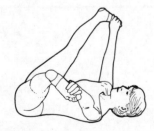

Sit with your legs outstretched in front of you. Put your feet as far apart as is comfortable, keeping the knees quite straight. With the spine erect, bend forward from the hips to grasp the ankles or toes. Exhale and continue to bend forward as far as possible, attempting to place your chin on the floor. Hold for ten seconds. Very slowly release and return to a sitting position. Repeat twice.

Effect: A posture difficult to perform in its perfection, the Bowing Down Pose benefits the entire body, making it very pliant. It is excellent for women, and also good for sufferers from haemorrhoids and urinary problems. It reduces the respiratory rate, thus inducing a calm state of mind and aiding concentration. This posture promotes a reverential attitude.

Caution: It is important to work very slowly and carefully towards the perfection of this posture, avoiding jerking and bouncing at all times.

The Partridge

Tittirâsana

Lie on your back. Exhale while slowly raising your legs overhead. Keeping the knees straight throughout, grasp your feet with both hands and separate them as far apart as is comfortable. Hold for ten to twenty seconds. Release the posture and slowly lower your legs.

Effect: The Partridge has a wholesome effect on the skeletal and muscular systems of the body. It imparts physical, mental, and spiritual powers.

Note: This posture is named after the small bird, Tittiri, related to the western partridge. The Tittiri is so powerful that it can overcome other birds four times its size. Legend relates that this little bird has not been smitten with excessive humility. It is said to labour under the delusion of being responsible for preventing the sky from falling upon creation. Hence it sleeps in this peculiar position, with its legs up in the air.

Bow Pose

As in Week Nine.

Triangle Pose

As in Week Three.

The Dancer

Natarājāsana

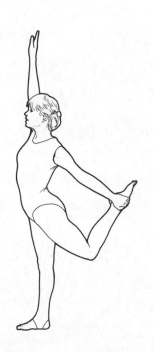

Stand erect, feet together. Shift your weight on to your right leg. Bend the left leg back and up, and grasp your foot with your left hand. (Check your balance and focus on a spot directly in front of your eyes.) Slowly and gently pull the entire leg up as far as possible. Raise your right arm high above your head. Hold this position for at least ten seconds, breathing slowly and evenly. Gently lower your arm and leg. Repeat the asana on the opposite side. Stand quietly for a few moments to observe the effects on the body.

Effect: Continued practice of The Dancer will increase pranic circulation in the body and raise the level of energy. The spine and the legs are strengthened, and posture and poise enhanced.

Note: Nataraj literally means 'King of Dance' or 'Lord of the Dance'. The posture is named after the great Eternal Being Siva/Sankara, the Profound Re-Creator, and is considered the basis of the Tandava, the magnificent cosmic dance of creation and dissolution which Siva performs at the beginning and the end of each cycle of creation. This dance, which Siva alone can enact, is deemed the most charming in all of creation and reflects the ever-changing flow of Nature.

The image of Siva Nataraj, the dancing Siva in a ring of fire, has become famous in sculptured masterpieces round the world.

Lord Siva is also regarded as the source of the entire system of yoga, the description of the 8,400,000 postures being derived from his instructions.

Breath Control

Complete Breath

Perform seven rounds.

Alternate Nostril Breathing

Perform seven rounds.

Relaxation

As in Week One or Week Two.

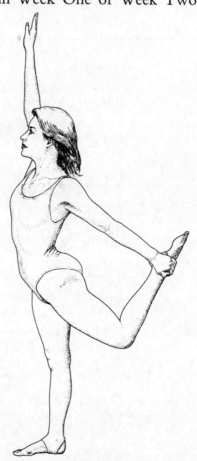

DANCER (Natarājāsana)

Meditation

During the previous week we have briefly referred to the *chakras*, wheels of energy situated at various points along the body, or more correctly, the subtle body. There are seven major chakras which correspond to different levels of consciousness. Before proceeding with this week's meditative exercise, it is important that you know a little about the nature of these energy centres.

1. The first chakra, the root chakra (Muladhara), is located at the base of the spine. Here lies the source of physical strength and stability. It is the seat of the survival instinct. Fear results from being stuck at this point. It governs the spine and bodily eliminations.

2. The second centre, the sacral chakra (Svadhistana), located in the lower abdomen, represents the expansive growth urge, instincts to maintain and preserve. This centre governs the entire reproductive system. Adverse qualities are greed, lust, and envy.

3. The third energy wheel is the navel chakra (Manipura), located in the centre of the abdomen. The sense of self-assertion and willpower manifests from this area. This chakra also governs the digestive system. Blockage at this point results in anger and digestive upsets.

4. The fourth chakra, the heart centre (Anahata), lies in the centre of the chest. Love, compassion, and humanitarianism are generated from the soul through this point. It governs the physical heart, the thymus gland, and the circulatory system. Blockage manifests in the inability to express heartfelt emotions and in disorders of the heart and circulation.

5. The fifth centre, the throat chakra (Vishuddha), is located in the throat area. Here verbal expression of higher knowledge, integrating internal and external realities, manifests. This centre governs the thyroid gland, the throat, lungs, and bronchi. Blockage results in disorder of the above, in difficulty in verbalizing, in stammering, and the inability to express feelings, resulting in a 'lump in the throat' sensation.

6. The brow chakra (Ajna), situated above the nose, represents the 'third eye'. It is linked with true wisdom, perfect intuition, and the power to see clearly

– clairvoyance. It governs the pituitary gland, the lower brain, and the nervous system. Detachment, asceticism, complete calm, and stability result at this level of vibration.

7. The crown chakra (Sahasrara), across the top of the head, is also referred to as the Thousand-petalled Lotus. This is the seat of profound creativity, peace, and bliss. It is associated with the pineal gland. This is the centre of ultimate unity and enlightenment.

There are many ways of activating and balancing these centres to promote physical, mental, and emotional well-being.

We have spoken about the effect of sound syllables in Week Seven. In fact, the origin of all singing and chanting dates back to ancient vedic times when the intonation of certain sounds was known to produce a particular effect on the environment as well as on the organs and glands of the body. All ancient cultures were aware of the effect of sound and used it effectively in their rituals and daily life.

There is a simple method of balancing the energy centres of the human body. Begin by focusing on your breathing, exhaling negativities and impurities, and breathing in pure energy. After a few moments, repeat the following sounds as you visualize energy coursing through each chakra, one by one:

1st   chakra – SRING
2nd   chakra – HRING
3rd   chakra – KLING
4th   chakra – BHRING
5th   chakra – LRING
6th   chakra – SOHAM
7th   chakra – PURNAM

Repeat each sound slowly at least seven times while concentrating on the corresponding chakra. The sound will effect a purification of nerves and remove blockages in the circuitry which runs along the spine to the brain.

An alternative method for experiencing and balancing the chakras is by visualizing their qualities as one breathes slowly, sending energy into each centre and beyond into the next. It is best not to concentrate on one particular chakra, but to visualize energy flowing through, focusing the breath upward from the base of the spine to the top of the head – free-flowing. The idea is to open up the circuits, not to get stuck at any one point along the way. Maintain the thought that everything you need is within you.

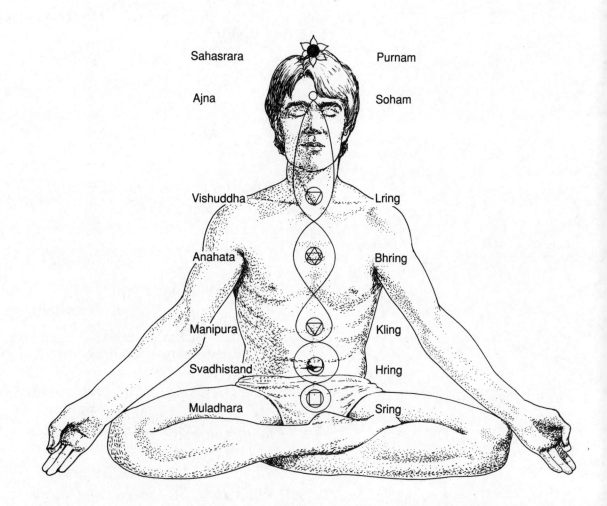

Sahasrara		Purnam
Ajna		Soham
Vishuddha		Lring
Anahata		Bhring
Manipura		Kling
Svadhistand		Hring
Muladhara		Sring

PERFECT POSE (Siddhasana) with chakras and corresponding seed mantra

Discipline and Practice

Nothing brings you into closer attunement with your fellow men and creatures, with their struggles and problems, than the heartfelt willingness to be of assistance where, when, and as the need arises. Making the resources of your abilities and understanding available to others not only benefits the other person, but also contributes towards your own learning.

The true spirit of service is a totally selfless attitude, not motivated by glorification and vanity. You do not force your help on anyone; instead you offer yourself as a tool, a channel for the natural flow of creative energy. It is this kind of attunement to the highest energy which begets the spirit and service of love. Abiding by its dictates, you will advance your own progress and upliftment.

MINDFULNESS

Mindfulness is emotional control
Mindfulness is coolness and clarity of thought
Mindfulness exists in overcoming emotional storms
By defusing them, rather than indulging them . . .

It is not being swept away
By fantasy and emotional distortions
Which are creations
Of faulty mental conditioning.

Mindfulness is being aware and conscious
Mindfulness is concentration
On the business of the moment.

Mindfulness is the dedication of
All one's thoughts, speech and action
To the Infinite.

WEEK ELEVEN

Freedom is a basic instinct in the nature of the human being. To realize this freedom it must be explored by all – without exception. True freedom is freedom of spirit and openness in the heart of every individual, in the spirit rising above all bounds into supreme consciousness. Indeed, freedom is the first condition of man's perfection.

– DR SVĀMI PŪRṆĀ –

Free will or destiny? This thought has been the source of much confusion. Confusion, however, lies in the question itself, which implies a choice. In reality there is no choice, for free will and destiny are ever linked and interdependent. One determines the other.

Freedom of will is a basic guarantee that has been bestowed upon the human being. Choice lies in its application. You have the privilege of exercising your freedom to build or to destroy, to shape your own destiny. This simple logic causes many problems. It places the burden at your own feet and makes you responsible for your own thoughts and actions. People find it much easier to accept terms like 'destiny' and 'fate' which generate the illusion of an outside agency bearing the responsibility, especially when difficulties and hardships present themselves. When all is well, the human ego will happily take the credit. Such thought only serves to thicken the clouds of misunderstanding and confusion.

To be aware of the meaning of free will and its obligations, to discriminate between what is helpful and what is harmful, and to be prepared to take full responsibility for your own thoughts and deeds, is to use your freedom wisely. Free yourself from the stranglehold of depression, anxiety, fear, and punishment. Use the gift of freedom as it was intended: as an instrument of evolution to enable you to grow physically, mentally, psychologically, and spiritually into a more mature human being. That task fulfilled, your true destiny awaits you.

Focus on Peace

Relax briefly and focus on the peace within you.

Warming-up

Lying down

Perform the stretching exercise, the leg lifts, and the pelvic twist.

Sitting

Perform the leg stretches, knee limbering, arm rotation, and the neck roll.

Standing

Perform the Woodchopper Swing.

Postures

Half-Lotus As in Week Eight.

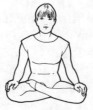

Half-Twist As in Week Nine.

Forward Bend As in Week Eight.

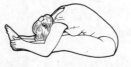

Inclined Plane

Katikasana

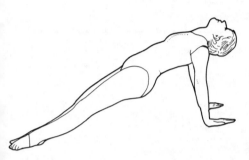

Sit with your legs stretched out straight. Place your hands behind you, either facing away from your body or towards your body, whichever is more comfortable. The arms should be perpendicular to the floor. Pushing your hands on to the floor, lift up the pelvis until the body is in a straight line. Slowly drop your head back and arch your body as far as is comfortable. Hold for ten seconds. Return to a sitting position and repeat twice.

Caution: This posture places a lot of pressure on your wrists, so be gentle with yourself.

Effect: The Inclined Plane, which is also called the Anterior Stretch, is a perfect counterpose to the Forward Bend. It revitalizes the spine and strengthens the wrists, arms, and shoulders. The heart chakra is stimulated, generating a loving feeling.

Stomach Lift

Uḍḍiyāna Bandha

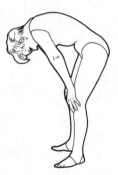

Before attempting this exercise, the bowels should be evacuated and the stomach should be quite empty. Early morning is, therefore, a good time for many people.

Stand upright, with your feet slightly apart. Bend forward a little, placing the hands on the thighs, just above the knees. Rest your weight on your arms.

Inhale, then exhale fully, expelling all the air from your lungs. DO NOT INHALE AGAIN THROUGHOUT THE EXERCISE. Now draw the upper abdomen inwards and upwards, creating a deep hollow. The lower abdomen remains relaxed. Hold until you need to inhale again. After a few normal breaths, repeat the exercise twice.

Effect: The Stomach Lift regenerates all the abdominal organs and strengthens the ligaments. It is especially beneficial for the stomach and intestines. Practised regularly, it will bring great relief to those who suffer from hiatal hernia, or prolapse of the rectum and womb.

Caution: Do not perform the Stomach Lift if you have ulcers. This exercise should also be avoided by women who have been fitted with an IUD (coil), as it is possible for the powerful contractions to dislodge the device.

The Plough

As in Week Six.

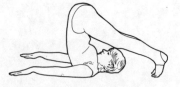

Shoulder Stand

As in Week Five.

Breath Control

Complete Breath with Chin Lock
As in Week Three – perform seven rounds.

Alternate Nostril Breathing
Perform seven rounds.

Relaxation/Visualization

Infinite Ocean
Lie down and allow your body to relax. Breathe slowly and evenly and quieten the mind. Remember that the mind and the breath are closely connected. Know that all is well. You are safe and secure. All your needs are taken care of . . .

Now visualize yourself lying on a beach. Make it the most beautiful beach you have ever seen. Notice the colour of the sand and the clarity of the water. Slowly walk down to the water . . . go in to where you feel comfortable and lie down and float on the water. Allow the water to support you entirely. Allow the motion of the water to lull you and to comfort you. Relax totally into the water, knowing at all times that you are completely safe . . .

Now allow yourself to go under the water. Imagine yourself swimming effortlessly, as though the water were your home. You can breathe as easily as though you were on dry land. Swim around and explore all the pretty rocks and plants you see . . . look at the many fish swimming past you. You are at home here. You feel safe and secure . . .

Now float to the top and let yourself rest on the water again. Feel the rhythmic movements of the waves as they carry you and become one with your breathing. Let your awareness expand and blend with the waves until you have become one with them . . .

Observe the spray that flies into the air, then filters down mistily to rejoin the waves. Watch how free it is and how easily it gives of itself, knowing that no harm will come to it, knowing that it will return and become the wave once more. Visualize yourself being as free and unconcerned as the ocean spray. Trust the universe to take total care of you . . .

The sun is overhead, shining warmly . . . and all about you are the reflections of the sunlight on the water, like tiny suns, unique lights unto their own selves that dance and move with the motion of the water . . . Allow your body to extend itself further over the ocean surface. Stretch out, and let the lights that are dancing over the surface dance over you, as your body and the surface of the ocean blend and merge . . . Feel that you have become millions of tiny, sparkling lights . . .

Slowly and gently begin to pull your body back together, leaving behind any distress, soreness, or disease. Very gently your body takes form again, floating once more on the surface of the ocean. Now you may place it carefully on the beach again. Feel the sand beneath you and let it run through your fingers. Stretch out in the sunlight and absorb the light of the life-giving sun. Then slowly let the scene fade from your mind . . .

Become aware of your breathing, and of your body lying on the floor. Slowly begin to move your fingers and toes. Stretch your arms above your head and give your whole body a nice stretch . . . relax . . . and when you are ready, slowly open your eyes.

Discipline and Practice

We have almost come to the end of our twelve-week course of Balanced Yoga. Just for a moment turn back to the first page of this book and carefully re-read the ancient Sanskrit Poem, *Look to this day*. It is always today, and today is your day of action. Regrets over the past are useless, as are fantasies about the future. Today is the reality you can do something about, today you can act.

At the beginning of this book it was suggested you keep a diary, making notes of daily events and recording your reactions. Do you relate hopes and fears on paper to be analysed later? Do you list your disciplines and goals, note your successes and failures? A diary can be a most valuable implement of self-help – a simple, yet effective method of getting in touch with yourself and releasing built-up tensions. It can help you discover your virtues and your weaknesses, thereby reducing confusion of thought and emotion.

Speaking in terms of free will and destiny, a diary serves as a documented check on the way you exercise your free will – and on its manifestation.

WEEK TWELVE

Yoga is like a huge, majestic tree that stands for expansion of heart, mind, and Self. Rooted in Nature, it branches out into innumerable realms of creativity, blossoming with bliss and the fulfilment of all human potential.

— DR SVĀMI PŪRṆĀ —

During the last eleven weeks you have explored the benefits of mindful physical exercise, and observed the effects of breathing techniques combined with guidance of consciousness into the various parts of your body. You have also subjected yourselves to some simple disciplines and opened your mind to positive, stimulating thought and experience.

The symbol of the tree with its strength and expansion also applies to the way you approach your learning. The blossoms of knowledge can only ripen into the fruit of attainment by the process of application and continuing, steady practice. The German poet and philosopher Goethe once stated: 'After all our learning, we only acquire what we put into practice.'

The criterion of yogic achievement is not how much you can twist yourself into the various postures, but rather how well you can apply the most simple posture, technique, or thought to the needs and circumstances of your daily life. With mindful practice, you can keep the body in good working order for its full life span – a fitting vehicle to carry you into realms of increased creativity and fulfilment.

Warming-up

Choose any warming-up routine suitable to yourself.

Postures: Juti Rupakas

Juti Rupakas consist of a combination of postures which flow into each other without pausing to relax. Slowly and gently the body glides from one posture into the next. Such postures are panaceas for the attainment of physical fitness, mental stability, and harmonious integration of the whole being.

Salute to the Sun

As in Week Seven.

Flowing Strength

Ṣakti Sanchar

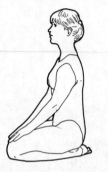
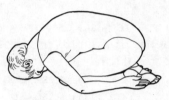
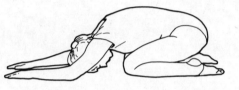

1. Sit in the Adamantine Pose for a few seconds, breathe slowly and focus on the solar plexus just below the breast bone.

2. Slowly bend forward into the Pose of the Child (also referred to as the Closed Leaf Pose), resting your arms by your sides.

3. Continue in slow movement to open your knees a little and stretch your arms and upper body forward into the Open Leaf Pose.

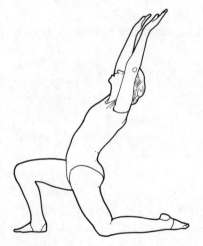
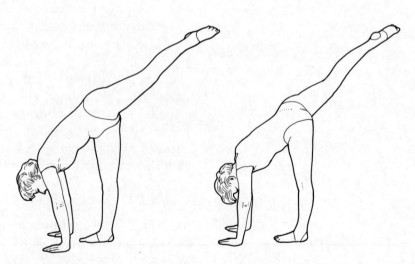

4. Shift your weight forward on to your hands and place the right foot just behind your hands. Shift your weight on to the left knee, raise both arms up high, and bend backward into a stretching salute.

5. Bend forward again and place your hands in front of your right foot. Raise your hips and straighten your right leg. Lift the left leg as high as you can. Hold this pose for ten seconds.

6. Change legs at this point by lowering the left leg and balancing on the left foot. Now lift the right leg up and back. Hold for ten seconds. Please make sure that the supporting leg is straight.

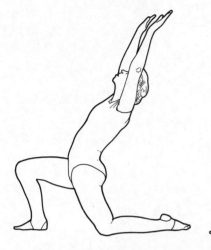

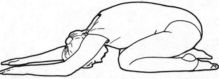

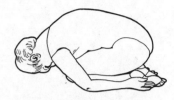

7. Lower the right leg into a kneeling position as in step four. Shift your weight on to the right knee. Lift up your arms and bend the upper body backwards.

8. Pull the left leg back into a kneeling position. Bend forward into the Open Leaf Pose, stretching your arms out in front of you.

9. Close the knees and pull your arms back to lie by your sides in the Closed Leaf Pose.

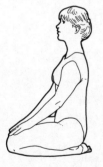

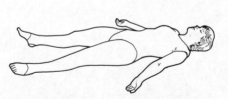

10. Slowly unroll your body and return to the Adamantine Pose.

11. Stretch out the body completely and relax in Savasana, observing the changes in your body.

Effects: This combination of asanas gives flexibility to the entire body and stimulates all the chakras. It promotes strength and a general feeling of well-being. Negative psychological patterns, such as fear and anxiety, are relieved, and the emotions are stabilized.

The Mighty One

Indra Jūti

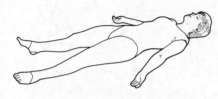

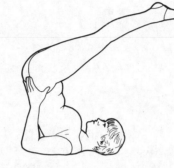

1. Lie in Savasana, the Relaxation Pose.

2. Smoothly move into the Inverted Pose, Viparita Karani (Week Two). Hold for ten seconds.

3. Stretch out into the Shoulder Stand (Week Five) and hold for ten seconds.

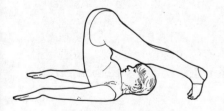

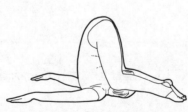

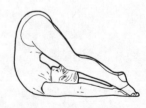

4. Let your feet move over and down into the Plough Pose (Week Seven). Hold for ten seconds.

5. Remaining in the Plough Pose, relax your knees and drop them next to your ears. Fold your arms loosely over the inside of your knees. This is the Spider Pose. Hold for ten seconds.

6. Straighten your legs behind you again and rest your toes on the floor. Stretch out both arms above your head to touch your feet. This is the Stretched Bow Pose.

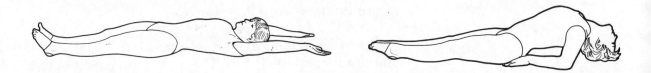

7. Slowly and smoothly raise your legs off the ground behind you, bring them forward over the head and gently lower them to the ground.

8. Move into the Fish Pose (Week Five), hold for ten seconds, then lower your body and rest.

Effect: The Mighty One builds physical strength and resilience as well as mental and emotional balance.

The smooth transition from one posture into the next may take a little practice but is well worth the effort. Juti Rupakas provide relaxation during active movement.

Breath Control

Complete Breath
Perform seven rounds.

Bumble Bee Breath
Inhale fully, filling the lungs from the abdomen. During exhalation, make a humming sound with your lips closed. Do five rounds. This will let the breath out slowly, resulting in better breath control, and stilling the mind in preparation for today's relaxation and meditation.

Relaxation

Choose any basic relaxation as in Week One or Week Two.

Meditation

During the relaxations and meditations of the previous eleven weeks, we have focused on peace-inducing images and on balancing the body, mind, and emotions. Today you are being introduced to a meditation that can help you attain further peace and stability – it can also transform your life. By deprogramming the negative conditioning of past thought and experiences, you will open the way to identification with what you really are.

In Sanskrit the syllables *So* (meaning He, It or That) and *Ham* (pronounced 'hum' and meaning I Am), combine into *Soham* – I Am That. This statement refers to the Divine in each of us, to the real Self. *So* is also the sound we make during exhalation, and *Ham* is the sound made when air fills the lungs. Whether consciously or unconsciously, all creatures repeat *So-ham* with each breath.

In our final meditation we will adopt the attitude of identifying with the qualities of the Self in totality, rejecting all else. You will 'wash' your consciousness of all the negative roles and concepts you encounter, and endeavour to be positive and attuned to your Higher Self.

Attunement

Begin by focusing on your breath for a few moments. As you breathe out, silently repeat 'So', and each time you breathe in, 'Ham'. Continue this breathing pattern each time you repeat these two syllables. For the other repetitions during this Attunement exercise, simply return to your normal breathing rhythm.

So – Ham . . . So – Ham . . . So – Ham . . . (seven times)

I am pure . . . I am blissful . . . I am happy . . .
I am not unhappy . . . I am not suffering . . . I am free from mistakes . . .
So – Ham . . . So – Ham . . .

I am the Infinite . . . I am the Limitless . . .
I am not small . . . I am not confined . . . I am not finite . . .
So – Ham . . . So – Ham . . .

I am total . . . I am whole . . . I am complete . . .
I am not the body . . . I am not the mind . . . I am not the senses . . .
So – Ham . . . So – Ham . . .

I am the Immortal . . . the Everlasting . . . the Eternal . . .
I am not dying . . . death cannot affect me . . .
So – Ham . . . So – Ham . . .

I am Love . . . I am Mercy . . . I am Compassion . . .
I am free from guilt . . . I am free from sorrow . . .
So – Ham . . . So – Ham . . .

I am the unencumbered Spirit . . . pure consciousness . . .
I am not bound by addictions . . . I am not bound by attachments . . .
So – Ham . . . So – Ham . . .

I am Knowledge . . . I am Truth . . . I am filled with Light . . .
I am not ruled by doubts and fears . . . darkness cannot affect me . . .
So – Ham . . . So – Ham . . .

I live each day in the awareness of my Divine origin . . .
So – Ham . . . So – Ham . . .

As you work with this meditation, constantly repeating these affirmations to yourself, you should aspire to live with these ideas and merge into *that* consciousness so that you may truly realize who and what you are.

Remind yourself that Divine Creative Energy is in all of Nature, including you. Be aware in every thought and action you perform that you are expressing some particle, however minute, of the Infinite which works through you. An appropriate thought might be:

Let every moment of mine be creative and wise, let my breath be nourishing to my being . . . As I inhale cosmic energy, let my body and mind be purified, my mind become as sharp as a sword, and my knowledge become as vibrant as fire. Let all my aspects – cells, organs, and atoms – become uplifted so that this body and mind will serve to further my evolution. Then I will, with great reverence and gratitude, offer back what Nature has given me.

NAMASTE

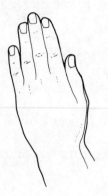

The traditional form of paying respect in Indian culture has remained as beautiful and meaningful today as it was in ancient days.

Placing the palms of both hands together in greeting is intuitively understood throughout the world as a gesture of peace and respect.

There is delicacy and profound symbolism in this simple gesture (mudra). The act of pressing the palms lightly together without space between them represents the firm and sincere heart which says: 'You are within me – as I am within you', thereby acknowledging the unity within all things.

To stand quietly for a few moments, with the hands in this mudra, is a pleasant and appropriate way of ending your yoga practice session.

GLORY BE TO THE ONE

Who is in the Fire
Who is in the Water
Who is in Plants and Trees
Who is in all things
In this vast Creation
Unto that Spirit
Be Glory

Upanishads